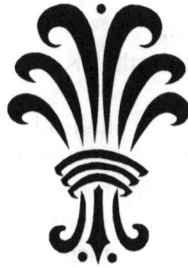

Holding

The Light.

By Jennifer Pickton

First published September 2008
By The Centre of Light, Letchworth. UK.

British Library Cataloguing in Publication Data

Pictures from Serif Image collection4 and Click Art. Royalty Free

Pickton Jennifer

    I.   Title : Holding the Light

ISBN 0955856914
EAN-13-978-0-9558569-1-4

Released for publication by
The Centre of Light, Letchworth.UK.
www.centreoflight.co.uk

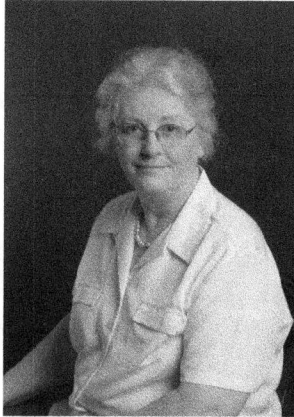

Jennifer Pickton.

In 1977 I joined a local Spiritual Healing group run by the late Pat Crocker who ran the Healers of all Souls. I was accepted as a promising Healer and introduced to alternative philosophies through the study of meta-physics, theosophy, meditation and psychology.

From 1978 to 1984 I wrote a series of 25 inspired verses which were an expression of my expanding awareness to release the deep seated knowledge within. In 2006 I started writing again and within a few months I had a volume of communicative dialogue from sources of Angels, Ascended Masters and Cosmic Lords.

I have established a connection to an inspirational source of a high order which is continuing to output interesting and constructive knowledge.

At the start of 2008 I developed some female health problems which resulted in the diagnosis of a malignant tumour. This book is the journey through the hospitalization period and the healing processes during recovery. I am having to put into practice all I know, to follow a spiritual healing regime.

I am a walking example of what spiritual healing can accomplish and as a channel for spirit my work is to spread this knowledge for the welfare and enlightenment of others.

Contents

Introduction

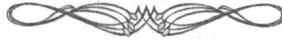

At the start of 2008 I had experienced a violent reaction to some medication I had been prescribed, which left me with a secondary infection for which three lots of anti-biotic pills failed to shift.

In February I suffered a haemorrhage and was referred to the Outpatients clinic at Lister Hospital, Stevenage, some three weeks later for an ultra-scan and consultation, but the clinic was running 2.5 hrs late. They did discover that the lining of my womb was thicker than normal which indicated some problem to be investigated further.

After another 3 weeks elapsed, it was April before I was seen at a special -fill in- clinic, where biopsies were taken from the polyps discovered within my womb. I was told that if irregularities were found I would need a hysterectomy.

This was the worst case scenario. I was also told that one of the polyps was misshapen, but not to worry, as the test results would come back in a couple of weeks.

During this time I went to visit my father who had just come out of Hereford Hospital after a stroke, and it was at my fathers home that I received the telephone call from my consultant, to tell me I did have a malignancy, so I would need to have the hysterectomy operation. I came back to Hertfordshire where I attended a MRI scan at the QE2 Hospital ten days later.

I had been told by my consultant that if I experienced any trouble between now and the operation, I should contact Ward 6 at Lister Hospital directly. I did experience some problems just before I had the MRI scan and that is how I spent two days at Lister Hospital under observation, where spirit was able to contact me.

On May 14th the Surgeons had their meeting and the next day I was contacted and told I would be having my operation on Friday afternoon 16th May 2008.

Ten minuets later I was again contacted by my consultant and asked if I could get to the hospital straight away for blood tests, as a 9.30am slot on Friday morning had become available. He suggested I take this vacancy, as most of the surgeons were going on holiday, which would leave a skeleton staff over the holiday period. This would delay the schedule of operations for another two weeks and I understood from him that urgency was advised.

Being of a practical mind, my first thoughts were, that to have an operation in the morning, was a much better option than in the afternoon, as the surgeons would be fresh and wide awake. This meant I would be the first on the days operating list. It also meant I didn't have to fast, as no food or drink by mouth was permitted for the twelve hours prior to surgery. My bags were already packed as I had anticipated events. From experience I knew that when things happen, they happen fast.

I had to psyche myself up to go through this unwelcome operation, as I had never had an intrusive operation before, and the only scar on my body was one inch long which I had received when a teenager. Like most people I am a coward when it comes to pain.

I had borne four children naturally and had never had any health problems until I reached middle age when I took Hormone Replacement Therapy (HRT). This kept me going when I needed to earn a living and provide for myself in all ways necessary, as I had divorced and suffered financially as a result.

This event changed my way of life and living considerably, but it did give me control and choice in my life, together with personal responsibility.

We are told that things happen to us in life for a reason and in my life I can pinpoint the occasions and events where my life has dramatically changed. I recognised that there have been cycles within cycles, which have required my attention to fine tune and bring about minor changes of direction, when one cycle has finished and another begins.

At this time in my life I firmly believe, that I am being prepared for an upgrade or transformation, and the physical removal of a tumour is the nugget of negativity which has accrued over the years, and is being eliminated in one fell swoop by this operation. This I have been led to believe, will enable my physical form to be of a lighter constitution, to enable the unity of my finer vehicles, which makes up the whole body of manifested form.

The reason for this is, so my physical vehicle can receive new and finer energies, for the purpose of communications from spiritual or cosmic dimensions hitherto new to channelled broadcasting. In addition I realised during my stay in hospital that there is a great need for healing services, as the present staff of both doctors and nurses are hampered by the red tape of current medical administration and policy.

Many of the nurses and doctors would do a lot more for their patients if they were given the time and encouragement to do so. I was greatly impressed by the dedication of those hospital workers who carry out a most valuable job of work in often adverse working conditions and environments. There are definitely Earth Angels of that I can assure you, who are operating in most difficult circumstances.

I felt that a mobile healing group should be formed and have deemed it a future aspiration of mine, to take a group of healers into the local hospitals, to attend those who are in need and would like healing, but are not mobile themselves.

Having been placed in the exact circumstances, I can now appreciate that when you are wired up, flat on your back and going nowhere, this is a time for the spiritual healers to get to work. Reducing operation trauma and fast tracking the healing processes can only be of benefit to patients and hospitals alike. Only time will tell if these ideas become realised. Action follows thought, so what we believe, can come true. I would never have thought five years ago that I would engage in writings of this sort.

The English language as a subject matter was never my strongest attainment at school, yet I am often given words of old origin or newly constructed, to suit the occasion. I do not have the kind of imagination that traditional story tellers have, so I am surprised at the things I write or am inspired to channel. What the future holds will be as exciting to learn from my personal viewpoint, as it will be, for those who read the published words I have channelled.

The following scripts and writings include the channelling which documents my journey from just before my operation and covers the recuperation time, with the many healings received directly or indirectly by both Spiritual healing and healers and Reiki healing sessions and practitioners and not forgetting those good thoughts and lighted candles from friends who hold traditional Christian religious beliefs.

It is possible that the content of these scripts will touch a nerve within others, who have undergone or who are facing similar circumstances. It is evident from the scripts that my guides the Crusader and Sister of Mercy are very close by, for which I am truly thankful, and can only marvel at their communications to me during this time and the calibre of the information imparted.

People are individuals and each life is unique, this is true, but we can learn many things from the experiences of others and the more we learn of what happens behind the scenes, the greater respect we may have for those spiritual beings that devote their life existence, to better the life and living of incarnate humans.

My own experience of life and living continues with its connections to health and healing of self and others. May this book provide insight and inspiration to bring to you, the reader, your own awareness and a point of spirit recognition, so you also can register the help that is given from the etheric realms, from those who shine their love and light of goodness, in service to the Lord Most High, that being of energy and light we call GOD.

Whatever personal beliefs may be held, it is a fact, that there are spirits who work hand in hand with their physical human counterparts. If we all had the ability to see and be aware of our helpers in spirit, then many of us would not struggle so hard, knowing we have unseen friends and colleagues to rely upon.

For all those who are aware of the spirit influences, know your trust and faith is well founded, as many healing agents are willing to work with us, if we allow it and give our permission.

The law of Free Will means, that humans must exercise choice. When acknowledging the spirit realms and all the influences imparted to us from that dimension, it is amazing how our life expands and blossoms.

It is the richness and wonder of spirit that brings light and sunshine back into the living physical life, when that normal life glow has be subdued by earthly and material events, and then receives revitalisation which takes on life anew, and brings into the now, that life of more abundance.

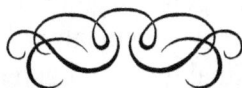

Preface

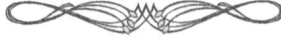

I had been visited by the cancer liaison nurse while at Lister Hospital who had come to talk to me about Radium treatment. At the time I was somewhat immobile and really didn't want to know about something planed for the future, as I was struggling to raise my energy levels to overcome the surgery aftermath, which had left me with an infection to battle.

In addition, the moment I was told about follow up Radium treatment, the word 'Barbaric' kept going through my mind. I knew that I would not survive such treatment, but I was resigned to the fact, that if it was absolutely necessary I would have no choice.

The nurse was understanding after I told her, I was not strong enough to deal with any further treatment, until I was healed from the operation and was up and about again. She did however tell me the criteria that the doctors used, in recommending Radium treatment to their patients.

She had brought a booklet with her for me to read, but she took it away again as I had no intension of reading it. I knew it would frighten me, and cause me to worry. She told me that when the laboratory released their findings and found out the extent of the cancer, that would determine if the cancer cells had gone past the half way measurement point of the uterus wall.

If the cells were within this limit, radium treatment would be optional. If the cells had gone beyond the half way point then radium treatment would be mandatory, as cells could have migrated beyond the original growth organ or site.

After my operation, the surgeons had come to visit me in the ward and had told me that the operation had been successful and that visually there had been no signs of spread in the ovaries or surrounding organs.

I hung onto what the surgeons had told me, as it was the most optimistic viewpoint and I continued with my daily ministrations of healing meditations and sound therapy. I had taken a radio/CD player into hospital and a number of CD's to play, to aid my recovery, as I knew I would not have enough self motivation or discipline and would need additional help and aid.

I don't think I have ever been so immobile or lacking in energy in all my life, so the period of hospitalization was for me an enforced rest, as the knock to my physical system was indeed great and profound.

I left hospital after ten days. I could have been discharged three days earlier but my wound was open and leaking, so when the ward doctor said I was fit to go home, the nurse said she would not let me go home because of the open wound. The Whitsun bank holiday loomed, so after a consultation the doctor suggested a compromise: a day home on sunday between 10am and 6pm.

This I accepted and was duly taken out to lunch, and then I watched some television to be returned to the hospital about 5.30pm. The exertion of that day was enough to shatter me. I fell asleep and woke up three hours later. It proved that I wasn't as well or as full of energy as I had thought, so I knew that in the time ahead I would be sorely tried and tested.

About ten days later, which was three weeks after my operation I was contacted by Lister Hospital to attend the clinic on the following day. The secretary told me I would be seen at 2pm even though an official appointment had not been made, and in effect I would be jumping the queue. I was told to report to reception and tell them of my appointment as this arrangement was with the consultant direct, who wanted to see me.

This worried me. I cancelled a previously booked appointment at my own doctor's surgery as it had been made clear to me, that it would be in my best interests to attend the hospital appointment and see the surgeon. This did not bode well. I became agitated. I started praying. I went to the clinic with a heavy heart.

After waiting for the hospital staff to fetch my records which were upstairs and not at the ground floor clinic, I again met my surgeon and the cancer liaison nurse with her radium booklet in hand. It was confirmed that the cancer had been an aggressive sort and not the type that they usually find within the uterus. I was told that I was clear of any spread to the ovaries. The other organs they had visually inspected and taken biopsies from, had also registered clear.

However, my surgeon recommended I visit Mount Vernon for radium treatment and he informed me, that he had already written for an appointment, to the Consultant Professor who was the leading EXPERT. Hence the nurse gave me the booklet she was holding and I was told I didn't need to see the doctor again until after my follow up treatment.

I was not very happy, but this situation was not entirely unexpected. I did ask for my wound to be dressed as the appointment I had cancelled had been with the nurse at my local surgery. It was fortunate that Sister Elizabeth was on duty at Ward 6A that day, so I was able to thank her for her administrations during my hospital stay, as she placed an iodine patch to my open wound. She called it her magic dressing.

My appointment to see the consultant professor at Mount Vernon was made for Monday 23rd June some three weeks later. I was not looking forward to this meeting in anyway. The journey was particularly gruelling as the M25 had been heavy with traffic and the thought of doing this everyday for five weeks did not appeal to me either.

In the waiting room there were people who had started cancer treatments in various states of emotional distress. One lady came out of her consultation in tears at what she had been told. This was upsetting. I was getting agitated again.

My name was eventually called and I was ushered into a consulting room. I had to wait another ten minuets before the professor arrived. A very sparse room decorated in yellow and blue. This was a very functional room with a table, two chairs and an examination bed. Clinical, was the word to describe the setting. I needed to calm myself so I shut my eyes and asked for help. I was immediately aware of two or three entities around me. One wore clothes of gold and seemed to envelope me with this colour so I was calmer. 'All will be well', went through my mind. I thought I sensed my Nun Guide and someone else with her, but I could not maintain the connection as the professor arrived.

Very matter of fact he introduced himself and opened my file. Well he said, I supposed those at Lister Hospital have discussed the matter with you and told you all about your case? Well I said, not exactly everything, and went on to tell him all that I had been told. He then disclosed information I had not known. He classed me as a borderline case as my cancer had measured 14 centimetres out of a maximum of 32 centimetres, so I was just within the half way point.

I was told that the operation had eradicated the offending material and given me an 85% chance of survival. The radium treatment was offered as a belt and braces exercise, but it was up to me if I thought it would be beneficial. He stressed that the side affects could be severe and I could land up with permanent damage to my bladder and bowel. The radium treatment would give me another ten percent added life expectance at best.

Something did not add up. What life expectancy? No one knows how long you are going to live. Even the best clairvoyant cannot make an exact prediction so far in advance. This information all seemed contrary to the information I had been given many years ago when a student. I had been told I would live a long life and more recently have been given direct instructions about future work and direction.

I reasoned that if I was optimistic and lived another thirty years, another ten percent would only give me an extra three years of life maximum. Against having treatment and thirty years of infirmity if I landed up with permanent damage, was a choice I considered, was certainly NOT a good one to make.

Spiritual healing will give me more than ten percent extra life expectancy, of that I am sure, so my choice is to have twenty seven years of good living, and rely on spirit and spiritual healing, to aid my recovery and steer me true.

It appears that the medical staff from Lister Hospital had covered themselves and had delegated the decision making process. I felt relieved. I thanked spirit. I was thankful to be alive and free. Free to choose how I lived my life and free to accept future options on life opportunities.

The professor gave me two weeks to make up my mind about having the radium treatment and told me to speak to the Marie Curie nurses at the Marie Curie Centre, before I made my mind up. This I did and was told by one of the nurses that the professor was highly regarded as 'The Expert' and what he recommended was the right choice to make.

In my case the professor had NOT made that recommendation. He had emphasized that it was **my personal choice**, as the advantages were questionable. He told me everyone has adverse cells floating around their body and it is the luck of the draw, if any should deposit themselves at a specific sight within the body.

I had been lucky, as the placing of my cancer had been in an area where the removal of an organ would not disadvantage me to any significance, as I had reached an age post menopausal and had discontinued hormone replacement therapy some two years previously. This meant there would be no post operative problems with regards to hormones which would be the case in someone pre-menopausal.

I could now start to live again and concentrate on the healing process, which I knew would be more complex than just the physical aspect of returning my body to normality.

My healing continues, both in body, mind and spirit. Life continues, with expectations and anticipation. Around me is doom and gloom from those around me privately, and from the general media, but I don't allow this to affect me.

I have insulation. It is my new suit of armour, my new protection, my cloak of blue light. My mediumship had been based on faith but now I know without a shadow of doubt that what I believe, I know to be a living reality and the knowledge imparted through me by spirit, is not to be dismissed.

The presence of Angels and Spirit Healers has been verified by other mediums who have not known my circumstances, yet through their own spirit guides are able to recount actual visits of spirit personnel to me during recent times.

I look forward to new work and new endeavours, knowing that failure is a mark of trying, and achievement and success is the result of having sufficient faith not to give up.

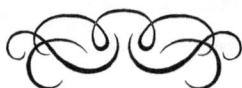

Chapter 1

My Guide the Crusader
30/04/08

I am your Crusader, come to talk with you.

We will keep you safe so do not worry over physical conditions as these will be put right. The changing vibrations affect body parts at their most vulnerable, so it is to be expected that a little aggravation will ensue.

Bring down the purple light and diffuse it with yellow – this brings the pink ray of universal love into play, and will help ameliorate the condition, so you can operate at this time effectively.

The lines of energy are being pumped up to greater heights and you will find plenty of energy on the morrow. The sun shines brightly on the righteous and this is your time of doing things right to appease those around you.

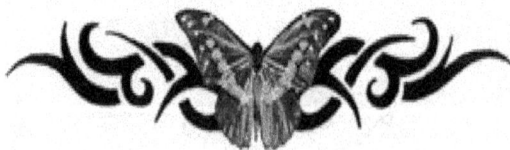

Chapter 2

The Scribe
01/05/08

In a middle eastern country where the sun shines hot both day and night, it is a welcomed event when you are invited into a cool courtyard of a scribes residence, located centrally within the city gates where the amalgam of humanity dwells. Here the chimes of Islam are heard together with the bells of Christian churches nearby. This is a place where all faiths reside, for truth dwell within the heart of each man, irrespective of his chosen manner of worship. Our scribe is a Christian who has lived with multicultural neighbours since childhood and no longer sees others as of different beliefs, but welcomes the opportunity to share insights of truths as his understanding allows, and can be used by all peoples, anywhere and at anytime.

Truth is the highest religion for it has no restrictions, dogmas or creeds. It is what it is. Truth is Truth. The truth may vary from individual to another individual as a man's perspective may vary from one to another. This is why spiritual teaching can be given, to awaken a deeper consideration when following a process of self discovery, as well as trying to find answers for life and living in the physical world you find yourselves in.

Humans are asking about the other dimensions of existence. They do not argue whether the many dimensions exist or not, for most take it for granted that there are other dimensions, because they either just know it is so, or they have experienced such, only to find that they cannot remember or hold the image as it was lost, just like a dream is forgotten.

It is not until another poses a reference to undisclosed knowledge, hidden within the deepest recesses of our minds, that we can recall as knowing, the simple truths exposed for our consideration.

Our scribe sits within his compound where a fountain is providing a calm and pleasant visual and audible background. This provides the sound vibrations to aid his thoughts and ideas, so he can formulate tonight's topic of inspiration.

Hello my friends, it is nice to see you again.
Please be comfortable.

I wish to take you on a short journey at eventide, when the first stars become visible in the night sky. The air is warm, the sky clear and the moon sheds light upon the area, so that much can be seen in the twilight. Scents from the flowing shrubs and trees, pervade the atmosphere to give a sense of comfort and well-being. Students are gathering together and sit upon rocks which provide seating, as they expect a learned holy man to speak tonight.

My friends, when I was young I was always eager to find answers by searching frantically and asking all those I knew. I expended much energy and did not receive the answers I sought, but found more questions were posed than ever before. Now I am older, I relax when I have a question and ask those in spirit to assist in the relay of answers. To do this I attune by saying prayers, so I may open up the channel of communication to those who are my guides and helpers, part of my spiritual family not presently on earth, but not far away from the earth vibrations. This is how I receive the words to relay to those who come to listen, to see for themselves how this method of communication works.

My friends, within each heart can be felt a heartbeat which confirms the living existence of the one who inhabits the form. If you can tune into others, to listen to their heartbeat, you will find the inner orchestra of beings, all sounding their notes and giving their experiences in a personal tune or sound, so that the merging of all the heartbeats will bring a truly significant crescendo to awaken those who do not yet realise that to be alive is to become aware.

How can you understand the mystic arts if you do not have the awareness to open to other dimensions of life and living? It is the discovery of your personal awareness that opens the doors to other dimensions and allows your soul to fly free in its own sphere of kin, to further your experiences and awareness. The light worlds beckon the celestial traveller as the gates of ascendancy are opened. Into the real world of galactic expansion and discovery you are propelled, and in transit you experience an elevation that feels as if you have floated away to sublime euphoria.

As your sight adjusts to the new vision of a celestial sphere, you marvel at the great sea of colours as the waves of coloured ribbons cascade upon the shores of white pearl sand. The pearl light moons from this dimension cast their luminescence upon the landscape and you can see the mountain tops in the distance as glass peaks. The landscape appears undulating as great swards of cornfields can be seen wavering in unison to the flow of coloured ribbons cast by the celestial seas. The rhythm of movement of life and living is one of gentle flowing above the colourful movement, to assemble at a temple located midway on a mountainside.

Elevated some distance from the lowlands, the vista spreads far and wide, so that the rhythm movement can be truly appreciated and heard, as music permeating the atmosphere and becoming a vibration of a most exhilarating force. As living forms unite, they generate more light and power into their surroundings, so that the tempo of vibrational living is accelerated to a higher pitch. The Angelic songs can be heard and visitors from the higher realms can come to meet and exchange ideas and knowledge in the Halls of Learning.

Many students assemble at these meeting places, which connect to other dimensional spheres so that universal knowledge and truths can be transmitted simultaneously. Many souls join the students of learning during the sleep state, so each consciousness can absorb on its own level. This way many are able to access the Akashic records at times of need or enquiry or reference.

What are the Akashic records you may ask? These are the records of every living form, from all levels of existence. Each galaxy or sector of the universe has its own reference library where all the records of life and living are held for eternity. You could say that these records are held on memory light sticks as this is the only manner in which records of such magnitude could be assembled. In fact the records are as much multidimensional or inter-galactic as you could imagine.

You may wonder how this could be. Such is the simile to that of water droplets, which make up the oceans of your world. If each droplet contained a life history in time and space, then together the whole is representative of the celestial seas. The oceans do not have a past, present or future as all is and revolves in continuum within the life cycles of the vibratory dimension of existence. Such is the best analogy for Akashic explanations.

You have plenty to digest and absorb.......God Bless You All.

May all sleep well, to absorb the knowledge.

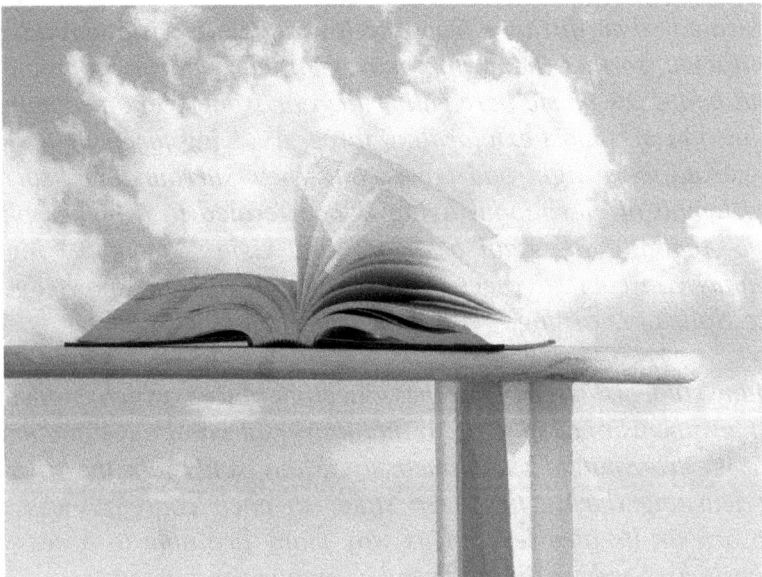

Chapter 3

Time of Concern
02/05/05

Your crusader draws near at this time of concern as you need to receive the reassurance that we in spirit will be with you to protect you and keep you safe. We have great plans ahead for you to relay our words and knowledge to bring to those your fellow humans.

Be not afraid of the physical malaise as this will bring you into a new era of health and vigour for you need the best physical form to undertake the work ahead. That which is not needed can be discarded. It is just an inconvenience or hic-cup in the forward flow of energy, taking place at present.

Many forms are adjusting to the New Age vibrations and as you know the opportunity will acquaint you with medics of earth to bring to them your own knowledge and both will learn to flow in wisdom. Bring in the healers by all means. Test out the system, so others may benefit from your example.

Hold the light. *Hold the dream. Hold the living life essence of your creator for he will be with you every step of the way. You are blessed and we will never let you down. Walk through fire and be unharmed for all is protected.*

Your work has just begun, so it is well to allow the physical aggravations to get out of the way now, so there are no impediments in the near future. A time for writing is ahead when we will furnish you with new material to while away the hours of recuperation. Your mind is ever active so use what you have to be able to bring about changes for better communications between all.

Your crusader is arming you with his silver armour so your protection is doubly assured. Hold out your hand and we will steer you straight. Trust in spirit as spirit places trust in you, for we are one and one is all. Sleep sound to energise anew.

----- 0 -----

A time has arisen to steer the ship through the choppy waters and direct the ship into a safe and calm harbour for a refit. The make over will be beneficial, so that the new version will be ultra fast and sleek in all its operations within all dimensions. The new technology installed will aid the receptivity as the radar scan will be able to connect with many channels for communications.

Extraterrestrials or light beings are eager to join with you, so you can open up the worlds of inter-dimensional levels that wait to be heard. Know that the Lord Creator is overseeing all the processes currently proceeding to generate change, so that the right conditions become available for spirit presence.

Allow the healing light to concentrate in the affected area.
This will bring some ameliorative assistance and allow any negativity to outward flow into the etheric regenerators, which are very affective at turning negative ions into the positive vibrations that can be used to create anew, on any level.

God Bless You.

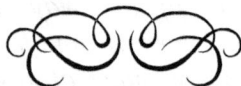

Chapter 4

Sister of Mercy.
05/05/08

My Guide.

Your Sister of Mercy draws near, for you have requested her presence to assist you in the time ahead. The vibrations of each of you are very similar and you can only register her nearness when quiet and calm. At such times the peace is felt and her group of administering Angels can also draw close, for all are helping to hold your vehicle in suspense, so that the form will remain buoyant and respond to the medical attention required.

Concentrate on your light vehicle since this is your most active form of operation. It is free from the impositions of the dense physical form and vibrations, and can manoeuvre freely and can at will, respond to the spiritual forces or energy. Steep yourself in the light and vitality will flow into your vehicle with a most welcome surge of upliftment. **Hold onto the light** *and you will see clearly the path of earth life before you.*

There are many that require your administrations, and to know what it is like to experience a spell in hospital, is like going through a transformational period. Many are altered when changes in routine are imposed. Most humans journey through life with certain expectations and when diversions happen, this is the time to question directions in the life and living. You may find you go off in a completely different direction after a thought provoking experience. This is because you have re-evaluated and your priorities have altered considerably. There is no reason in your case to change dramatically, only to understand that the work ahead is of a high order and you are being prepared now for the tasks ahead.

The many ordinary humans rely on those more able to help them, when they do not understand or do not know how to cope.

You have much teaching to give and the demonstrations of clairvoyant communication are a part of your medium-ship, demonstrating the connection between the dimensions, which make up the galactic super-highway. All are required to contribute to this great innovation of the present age. It is always difficult to educate those who seem uninterested. It takes a spark of interest to ignite the individual into realisation. It only takes one spark to light up an otherwise dormant form.

It is for you to find the key to each human, so they will respond accordingly. This happens when you give readings, as in conversation a subject is brought to the fore and the spark ignites right there before you. Tingling is felt in the recognition of spirit, so you know when you have activated another into recognition, by experiencing this feeling of confirmation. Your words must be published for the race needs the wisdom contained therein. Some will not understand, but many others will, and some intellectuals will analyse this and that and speculate on where the truth lies.

When the light of tomorrow shines brightly for the mass of humanity to see, then the many who are kind in heart, will speak out with their inner knowledge and understanding and the world will begin its major change. For change must occur to bring about a more considerate race of humankind. The seeds have been sown and are waiting for the fertile ground in which to spring forth into abundance.

The international scene for peace and enlightenment is gathering pace in all quarters. There are those who have money aplenty so the finances will be brought forth. Those who believe in a new age, a new era, will gladly give all they have to bring hope and prosperity into reality for their children's future.

Be aware of me in the peace and calm, and know that love unites us all, regardless of which world we inhabit. You have far to go in your life plan so do not waver in your belief for a bright future. Take care of today and the future will take care of itself.

Live for today and life will ever be surprising, for each day is a new dawning of Gods abundance and the more you experience, the greater is the understanding of all things. God bless you and know you are in safe hands for we are always near.

……… Amen

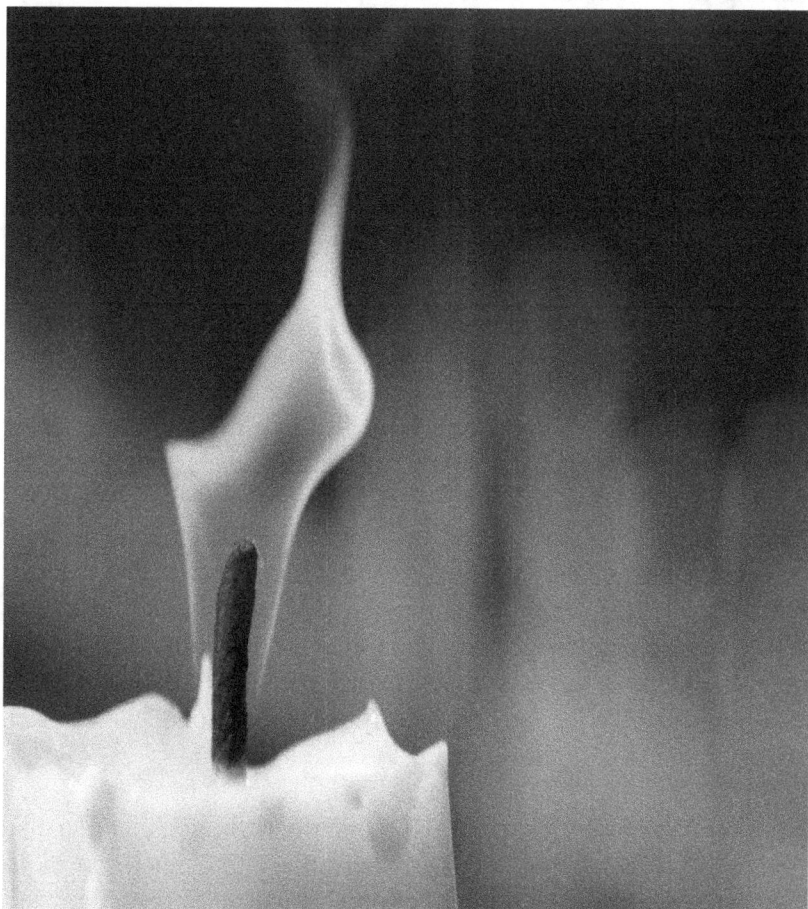

Hold the Light

Chapter 5

Earth Healers
05/05/08

Spirit dialogue:-

The Earth Healers can do much to assist the recuperation or restorative processes to the form and tissues at cellular levels by attuning to the healing guides and spirit doctors and nurses who assist the earth institutions, and provide stimuli to act. Many forget that to receive assistance both visible and invisible the request must first be given. Permission is needed to intrude into what is another's aura and space to bring about altered states, when rebalancing the energy centres, fields and physical form or cocoon. The healing team must stand by to act on demand, when the signal is given, so that synchronization of the applications and methods can take place.

The note must ring true, so a re-tune-ing takes place throughout the octave of being, and likewise the colour hues are re-vitalized and purified to shine clear and bright. When receiving a refit, or major refurbishment, the area in form, needs clearing and cleaning, to enable the free flow of energies to activate the mechanisms of animation and co-ordination. The mental state of the patient has a great bearing on the whole procedure as it acts like a dam or lock, which is either fully open or at various stages of closure depending on how positive are the affirmations and intent. Not everyone can adopt a totally positive attitude, so we in spirit step in to alleviate the faculty of the personal will, which wavers at the first hurdle it meets.

We direct the attention away to more interesting topics, so that there is little interference in the unconscious and super-conscious states, even if the conscious persona is fantasizing with itself. Gradually the sense of reason will prevail and the calm and peace of pure love will be felt, to act as the healing balm upon the one who is in need. Know that it is enough to give yourself over to the Loving Lord, your Father Creator, the Almighty. He will provide all that is necessary for your needs and will provide instructions to us his helpers and healers, as to what is the best and most appropriate action to give you, in your hour of need and personal attention.

We in spirit welcome a channel to relay our thoughts and knowledge. We seldom get the opportunity to speak directly to our patients as we have long worked incognito as is Gods way. As we draw nearer to the human race, we understand the need for individuality so we speak as one, although often we are a group of one mind, you understand? Many in spirit specialise in medical matters and treatments which are given as ideas or new techniques for humans to use and understand.

With modern technology the scope is widened to more non-invasive methods, but even this is but a phase, as the psychic surgeon is the one who can perform what you call miracles, with little or no after affects upon the physical form. When the knowledge is accepted about the healing energy, and how healing energy works, more will adopt the approach to use positive white light energy for healing.

The needs of those who do not have great physical wealth are the very ones who are using these methods of healing energy flows, and learning quickly that when groups gather for specific purposes, the energy of will, love and trust, evokes the healing entities and allows the God light into the midst, to bring about those instant cures and miracles you know and hear about. This is not some fanciful dream it is the next reality, for the medics of tomorrow must be versed in medical, electro-mechanical and spiritual expertise and know-how.

The spiritual expertise is based on the faith and surety that the energy of electro-magnetic properties will work, to alleviate the problems found by changing the faulty properties into the correct vibratory rate.

This is when the medic will know what vibration each major and minor organ of the body vibrates at. It will be significant if a given note is off-key, for that is when diseasments occur. It is then required to ray charge the area with the correct corresponding charge of energy (Light, Sound, Pulsation or Vibration) to affect the re-balancing to optimum health and function.

The laser light used at present can be widely used, as well as the sound waves presently used to disperse blockages. Sound has greater uses in the psychiatry fields and also in the rebalancing of auric energy fields of a patients light form. The advances in future years will incorporate more energy uses, so that it will be as a last resort, that the removal of tissues is performed to eradicate diseasements. X-rays of the future will be colour co-ordinated as digital technology takes centre stage and captures the faster vibrations of the ethers.

Ask someone to photograph patients in a hospital and see the power lines of the ethers exposed. We in spirit are working endlessly to bring about the regenerative box that will revolutionize the form structures rehabilitation to health. The healing box or capsule, (like a coffin - as it will look very similar) has been imagined in your science fiction, where a person who is injured is immersed for a time within the healing box and then resurfaces as new.

THE IDEA IS TRUE, so you should hold this image and the medical scientist should work towards making this a reality. All good ideas are filtered down into the accepted arts and viewed as fanciful, until such time when fanciful ideas becomes fact. What is really happening is that future happenings are pictured ahead of linear time, so the race can become acquainted with the idea and accept such, when the time is appropriate.

Many ills are as a result of life circumstances which cannot always be changed, so those born into a particular area are prone to certain ailments, because of the life style and cultural circumstances.

Natural disasters happen, and when a human is caught up in such events, damage occurs indiscriminately. It is a part of karma that you incarnate into a particular family, town, country or race. The life blueprint that you elected to undertake is given as a guide, with many variations. It is up to you to make your own decisions in life which will take you along your chosen course. You may not reach the goal you set yourself, but may have many other experiences along the way just as valuable.

To embrace the earthly day with optimism is a good way to start each day and each night it is good, to say thank you to your creator, in acknowledgment of the life you are living and all the blessings you have received. Any prayer spoken from the heart is the best way to converse with your spiritual connection and that way you can come to remember your sleep time excursions into the other worlds of existence and experience.

Many souls originate from outside the earth planet and come from other stars and universes. It is to your planet earth that such attraction beckons the many, to provide those opportunities for soul progression. When there is no fear of death, the soul is freed from its constriction within form and can manifest openly in the physical and etheric dimensions, showing its higher and lower selves united as one.

The glow of Gods love and light shines forth from that form as it has been liberated into its light being body. Now to demonstrate what is truly a spiritual person who can reside upon earth and function on the many other levels of existence. This brings into the physical manifested world the true love, light and beauty of the heavens.

In doing so, the earth world will respond in its transformation to a lighter vibration. The Christ vibration of love to all men.   - Brotherhood, Sisterhood, and Nationhood.

The earth will come to unite with the understanding, that its existence is reliant upon the universal Creator, the Great Omnipotent Deity we call GOD.

God bless you and thank you for relaying my words.
I am one from the White Brotherhood known as Lister.

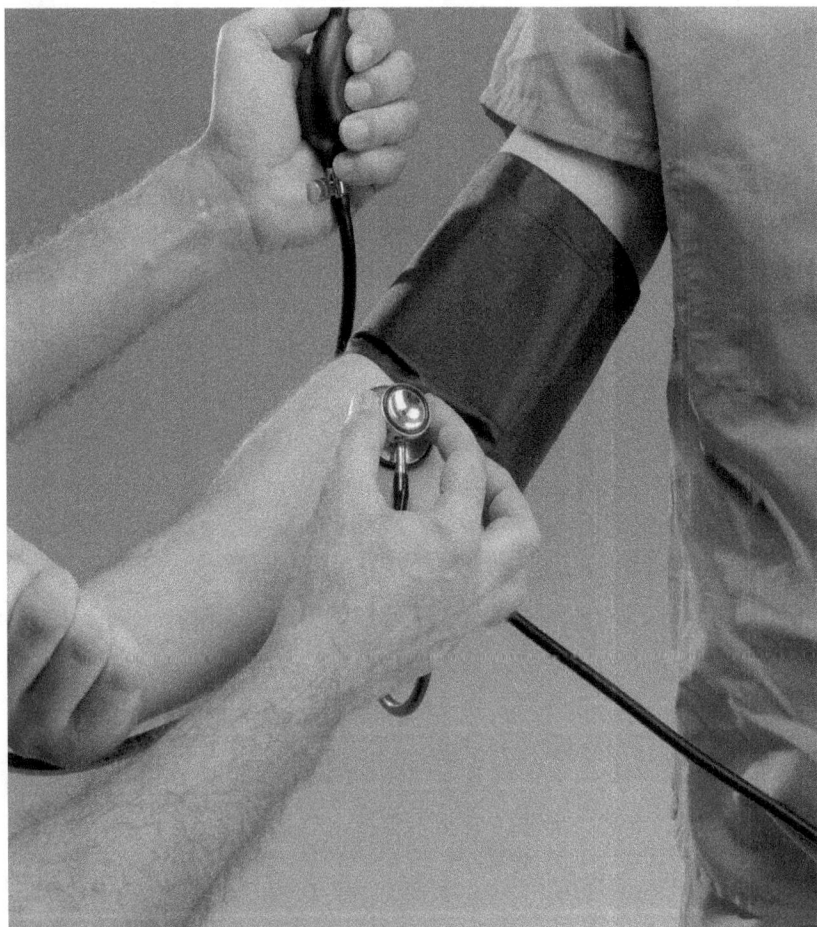

Listen to the Heart Beat

Chapter 6

Ward 6A
Lister Hospital, Stevenage, Herts.
08/05/08

I had spent the night at the hospital under observation as my blood pressure was very high and I was having problems with my female anatomy after I had been told just a few days prior, that I would need a hysterectomy due to a malignancy.

A young lady had been admitted about two hours ahead of me and was waiting for a bed when I first met her in the day room. By the time I had been seen to and got checked out, it was 11.30pm. I think the doctor felt sorry for me as I was the last to be seen and I had been waiting three and a half hours. I think also, the doctor was worried about my blood pressure as the student nurse couldn't get a reading (I had gone off the scale) and he was playing safe after hearing my recent story of events.

When I awoke the next day, the young lady who had taken the bed opposite to me was still fraught. We got talking about the National Health Service and alternative healing, and she told me she had undertaken a course for Indian head massage as well as a general holistic healing course. This conversation led to my revealing that I was a practicing Spiritual and Reiki Healer, and also a working clairvoyant Medium.

She told me, she had dabbled with the healing arts but didn't have time to follow any more therapies, as she was six weeks pregnant and was in for a scan to see if this pregnancy was ectopic. She had been having private fertility treatment, so was acquainted with the different standards within the various hospitals which she recounted to me. I registered that her grandmother was around her, so I was able to describe her.

She was a very hard working lady whose life had been one full of hard work and she had adopted the attitude in her life of taking what life threw at her and getting on with it. This was the main message to her granddaughter who was very much like her in temperament and looks.

The young lady had received messages from her grandmother before she told me, so was not shocked when I was able to relay the message to her from her grandmother 'to take what life throws at you and get on with it'. Three hours later after a scan she was returned to her bed. Somewhat in shock and surprised to have been told that the pregnancy seemed fine and was not ectopic. She was however, carrying triplets! The medics had told her she had some serious thinking to do, as she had the option to abort one or two embryos if this is what she wanted. It is not my place to make decisions for others, only individuals can make decisions for themselves in order to steer their life course. My comment to her was 'If your health is fine - three babies make an instant family' it is early days, so do not rush into making decisions in any haste.

In the afternoon when a new lady took her place I again engaged in conversation with the bed occupant. This was a lady in her seventies who was to have a cyst and ovaries removed. This lady was very fit as she takes long walks with her dogs and has done so for many years, which provides good exercise and fresh air for her general health and vigour. She was worried about the operation and its affects, as she had last been in hospital twenty five years earlier, when she had undergone a hysterectomy.

I explained to her about the chakras or energy centres of the body and the rainbow colours that bring the various colours and energies into our body form, to re-vitalize and uplift in times of need. I gave her instruction to imagine a white cloud above her head and bring this white light of pure healing energy into her body form to extend and expand its healing affects, so that her recuperation would be assisted by this additional uplift of healing power, at a time when she would be feel particularly low and vulnerable. I assured her all would be well.

The medics came to visit her pre-op to discuss an epidural and she turned to me for confirmation as to this being the right thing to do? I could only say to her, that it would be better to have more pain relief than not enough and she should go for it, if that's what the medics were recommending.

I thought it might be a good idea for me to have one too, when it was my turn to have an operation, so this event was a double sided consideration applying to both of us. On Tuesday 13th May 2008 I had an appointment at the QE2 Hospital to have a M.R.I scan. At 11.30am. My step daughter accompanied me to the Welwyn Garden City Hospital to keep me company. I was ushered in on time and fitted with an input vent in my left arm.

The nurse was very gentle and it didn't hurt, unlike the previous occasion when the same thing occurred at Lister Hospital six days earlier. While I was waiting for my turn in the doughnut scan machine, the radiologist came to have a chat and she commented upon the fact that I seemed very calm. I told her that I could not change what was to happen, it was up to me to get through it and concentrate on what came afterwards.

In other words I was concentrating on my recovery and not on the operation itself. We had a talk about healing and got onto the subject of reincarnation. She thought this subject was the terrain of the buddhist, so I told her, that it's all down to individuals what concepts they accept, to aide their personal pathway of spiritual progress and enlightenment. It seems that my journey through the medical maze of curative treatments is also an educational tour for those medical and ancillary contacts around me.

Spirits use every opportunity to activate the communicative function, to get the best help and advice across, to the point of where there is a need.

Life and living is truly a wonder if you have eyes to see.

Chapter 7

Lister Hospital 08/05/08
Father Ernest comes to call:-

I administer to all those who are in hospitals as I help those souls to connect with the healing Angels, to bring about and strengthen their connection to the spiritual sources, which provide the sustenance of will and purpose, so necessary in a patients mind and emotional vehicle.

The resolve to activate the self healing abilities within, and those agencies without, is necessary to start the healing processes.
Often in the trauma of illness or injury, the human will and motivations become lost in the activity of present experience and events. It is often in sleep time that I visit, so I can activate the mechanisms within each patient, to enable the individual to become internally aware, and thereby realise the need to use affirmations and confirmations of intent, to reinforce the mechanisms of healing.

When I was on earth, I dealt with mans soul and was eager for his salvation. I thought that it was through the church that mans salvation could be sought. I did not realise that mans salvation is through himself, when he becomes aware of his own spirit and acknowledges the connection to his spiritual Father, the Creator of all things.

I now know that each individual must find his own avenue to God by connecting his own spirit or soul to that of the Godhead. The church is there to act as a guide or teaching house to give purposeful directions to those who seek. Gods house is not some physical building, but the home for all his creations, which resides at the heart of each living thing. So look into your hearts to find that divine spark of God and when recognised, you will know and can experience that connection with your Lord Creator.

Often at times of hospitalization, the crystallization of desires and aspirations can be seen clearly, and when evaluations take place, it is a time to eliminate fear, so the purity of white healing light can act as a transformational remedy. When fear is eradicated, the doors are opened to receive the healing energies and there are no impediments to the free flow of healing power and light.

My ministry on earth was much different to what I now have adopted as my main interest and pursuits. To restore human souls to their elevated state in the kingdom of heaven, the various levels or vehicles of being need to be harmonized and balanced, so it is best to start while on the physical plane. When visiting a hospital, it is like visiting a church. It provides a time for realisation and direction, evaluation and appraisal, so that the life journey, the pathway of world experience can be consciously appreciated and assessed.

Not all people have to visit a hospital to achieve this realisation, but many do through disease or injury, which represents a crisis point in the life journey. By taking time out to attend to personal needs, the viewpoint is turned inwards for self examination. Not all people are spiritually aware, so I come to assist in the inner awakening, so a deeper understanding can be established. What many do not fully appreciate is that the healing Angels work within the corridors of the hospitals and healing centres.

Some are earth Angels and operate as present day nurses and doctors. You know these souls, as they have a dedication and calling beyond what is normally accepted. Their whole focus is towards their fellow human and they are often pioneers in medical matters taking the understanding of their profession forward to new levels.

A number of the White Brotherhood have served in the medical fields and bring illumination to those incarnates who are present day researchers and medical pioneers. Their influence extends further into the scientific and engineering departments, to bring to the medical profession a wider understanding of how interrelated are all areas of expertise, and how some in particular are revolutionizing the way modern surgery is carried out.

With robotics, electronics, electro-mechanical and magnetic applications, as well as light and sound therapies, metal, gem and crystal understandings, all have a part to play in the re-constitution and maintenance of the human form, to make up and house the physical, emotional, mental and spiritual bodies of the complete balanced and animated human being.

I find myself visiting the hospital chapels as many visitors use these places as a sanctuary, where they can send healing prayers to their sick and suffering relatives or friends presently in the hospital receiving treatments. Others are finding solace after a loved one has passed to the higher life, and others are patients themselves who are the walking wounded, who come to ask for help and healing direct.

I therefore administer the healing and spirit flows to deal with direct healing and upliftment, internal or remote healing is sent when energies have to be directed to another recipient from the source request. I do deal with those who come to mourn the passing of a loved one or friend, for this is an area of double requests, since the one who has passed is journeying to their allotted place, and I make sure that the lines of light are straight and true, so that the departed one is transported on a beam of light to his or her heavenly home.

The ones left behind are troubled as they face the earthly life without the direct influence of the one departed. Often there are unresolved issues which cause anxieties, such as not having said good-bye or not having said the very things that needed to be said. There is guilt, fear for the future and grief to be addressed. For both parties either side of the veil it is a period of adjustment.

The one who has departed has the best experience, as they enter into love and light and a rejoicing takes place at the reunion of souls, when relatives in spirit again assemble, to greet and welcome the new arrival. Those left upon the earth plane can be affected by denseness, darkness and depression as the physical separation of a loved one is felt in the mind and emotions. In acute cases there is utter despair, particularly if the transition was unexpected, and just like the one who experienced the physical trauma, the grieving relative or friend experiences the same traumatic pain which affects the emotional and mental bodies of their form.

This happening can have repercussions upon the physical form if left unchecked. The malaise can manifest as lethargic movements, the inability to connect with the physical world of which they are apart. It can happen that a withdrawal of the mental and emotions occurs and the bereaved becomes the aggrieved. Here is when great help is needed to understand the mechanisms of the relationships between the four aspects of human form.

There are many races which actively encouraged the wailing and outward expressions of grief. This is beneficial to the physical form, as it releases the grief into the atmosphere for it to disperse. Many therapists and physiologists work to alleviate repressed emotions and change mans thinking, so that a more positive and healthy approach can be adopted. This is the first stage of recovery when the awareness becomes self aware and positive steps introduced to overcome the blockages of mental and emotional origin, which require a cleaning and clearing out, so that the free flow of light energy can take place and the form returned to its optimum working state.

Know that as well as the many nurses and doctors that attend a hospital, the compound is staffed by many helpers of other disciplines and many volunteers. Amongst these are other Earth Angels who assist on a humane front in anyway they can. A patient's recovery is assisted by being freed from material problems and decisions, if it is known that someone dependable can deal with material matters, during the hospitalized period.

To be freed from immediate worry leaves the patients free to continue with self orientation and discipline.

Discipline is required of the self to provide motivation and upliftment, so energy can follow thought, and in doing so, the emotions can follow suit to affect the physical being, so you should feel a better alignment taking place, when given positive directives and thoughts towards recovering your optimum health.

Such is my ministry within the hospital of Lister. It is a large compound of diverse activity. I seek the calling souls and thank you for helping those around you to be positive in all that they think, say and do. It is nice to have helpers who understand the energy flows. I have sent you some white light also, for she who gives, also receives.

God Bless You

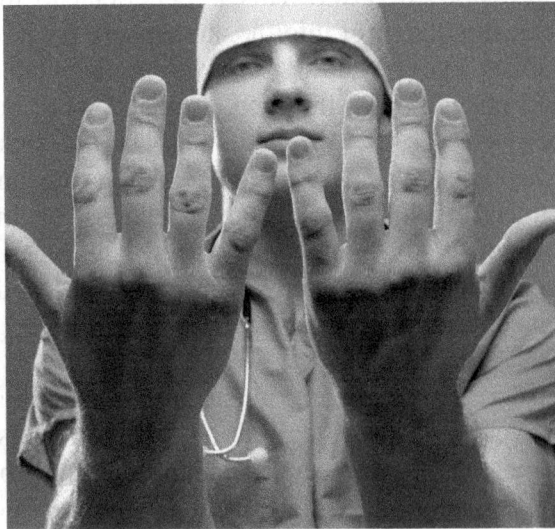

Healing Hands

Chapter 8

The Ghost.
Dedicated to Sister Elizabeth Saunders
Lister Hospital Ward 6A North
19/05/08

On the third day post operation, the ward sister came to see me. She had found out that I was involved in a spiritual healing group and announced that she had undertaken an Indian head massage course. She told me she had experienced some tragedy, as only last year, she had lost both her father and brother, who had died within eight weeks of each other.

She then informed me that they had a resident ghost of a lady who had appeared to some of the young nurses, in a room that was set aside for those who were ready to die.

Without thinking I began to give a description of the lady as she appeared in my minds eye. However the ward sister had not actually seen her, but she did not dismiss this phenomenon, as some younger nurses had been frightened by the encounter. I asked her 'who was Elizabeth?'... 'I am she said!'

I later confirmed the description of the lady ghost, from an Irish nurse who said she had seen this lady a number of times and also confirmed that the lady ghost always sat in a chair, in the corner of the room wearing a blue robe. (The colour blue is the traditional colour for healing)

Tuning in, I was able to receive the following information:-

'I am a lady who died at the hospital in 1987. I was in my seventies, quiet slim of figure with light grey hair that was straight and collar length. When I was younger I worked as a nurse and had to pin my hair back out of the way.

I nursed many ladies with female problems and I choose to help those presently suffering the same conditions, who attend this female ward and who are in need of assistance. I do help those who pass over. I became a matron and liked to take charge at important or major events. I often sit in a chair waiting for the patient's time of transformation, to ease their transition and on occasions, those on the physical plane have commented on seeing my presence. The young nurses of today are not trained or taught about the more subtle energies or vehicles of the physical form, and therefore are not so sensitive to the etheric vibrations which indicate the changing energy forms around and abounding.

The more mature nurses have greater experience and have dealt with much which is or has been considered unexplainable. They have greater empathy with all ages and have experienced life outside of hospital, to an extent that brings understanding of wider issues and problems a patient may have, in terms of practical living, existence and circumstances. There are many of us who walk the corridors of Lister as we use our skills as experts would, when administering their trade to the populace. There are so many people who enter and leave this hospital, with conditions dealt with and others overlooked.

Often a patient has to return each time the same problem surfaces. We in spirit could advise accordingly if we had trained clairvoyant and clairaudient doctors and nurses. Some are beginning to heed their instinct, their sixth sense, that intuition that tells them a certain something, which becomes instinctual knowing, so when they delve deeper within the patient's history and circumstances, an underlying problem may be identified, which can be seen and treated before it gets to a crisis point.

The dramas of a hospital are many and varied and it is important that those in the physical world can react, when we tap a shoulder or use some other indicative manner, to highlight the attention in relation to a particular problem. So to the new doctors and nurses, we ask that your awareness be fine tuned to the more subtler vehicles of form, that indicate our presence, and take advantage of the many services we can offer you, to make the practical health care function work to greater efficiency and effect.

Not all patients can be healed or cured it is true, but all can be helped and given upliftment. By administering to your fellow human, you are demonstrating love in action, and where love and light prevail, if it is combined with positive thought, energy will follow through to bring the healing power into effect, in the best interests of the one who comes in need.

God Bless You.

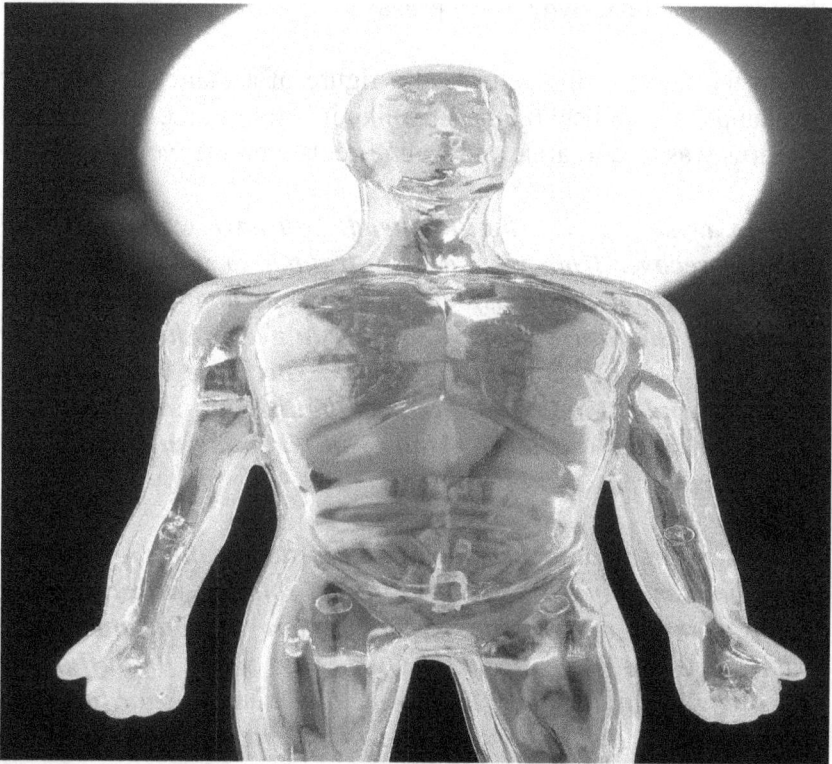

Chapter 9

Day Seven
Lister Hospital.
22/05/08

I awoke at 5.50am with my bones and insides aching from the nights deep rest and needed pain killers to take the edge off this acute discomfort. As I lay there waiting for the painkillers to take affect, I became aware of three nuns lined up along my right hand side. I then registered Angel wings at the foot of my bed and knew that healing was being administered from the spiritual realms. My temperature had retuned to normal after three days of treatment for an infection. I had a sudden urge to get clean, feeling as if I had sweated it all out during the night, and was now free from the fever which had prevailed.

From the Angel wings emerged a figure of a man who held out his hands as if to beckon me. Just like it is told in the Bible, when Lazarus was told to arise and walk, I registered the words:

Get up, arise and live the life ahead. You have work to do and need to recover from your earthly trauma so the healing rays can bring about the transformation to your bodily form that is needed for the future work. Many are in need of healing as you are fully aware and from your own experience you can now draw the understanding and respect that is your due. Many will listen and many will learn. Many will take note and many will benefit from your administrations.

We assemble by your bedside to administer healing to you. We have been running as a team of three, rotating with two other teams of three, making nine sisters of mercy at your attendance with the Great Angel Healing Guide who sends his influence. We are wielding the energies to keep the balance. Your form has undertaken a major blow to one of its energy centres, which provides the majority of life vibrancy to the other parts of your form.

In your case we have been substituting the sacral centre by channelling the terracotta rays into the void, so connecting the base centre and solar plexus, which makes up the lower triad, which acts to ground the form to the physical earth dimension. It is a question of finding a balance, so the energy centres can be re-aligned and adjusted to the new frequency. This will take a few weeks of your time as you heal. The new energy has been centred and will gather in force as you grow in physical strength and vigour.

The lighter finer energy will give you that quickening, to act as a springboard for the upper energy triads, so your communicative attributes will be reinforced accordingly, as the free flow of light energy is allowed to accelerate without any obstructions or curtailments, in the seven vehicles of your total body. The light vibrations are scintillating to a new clearer mauve, turquoise and gold. A new note, a new sound, a new tune or melody, to take you into the ascension of your being, as it merges with its light body, to manifest in two dimensions with added strength and definition.

The Christ light grows stronger and you respond well to this beautiful energy which brings love, light and wisdom. You are a teacher, so must spread the knowledge within, to all who will listen and to some who don't want to know, but need to know for their own future awakening. Gather around you a band of helpers and we this side will match like for like, to bring about that mobile healing unit that can and will make a difference to those in need.

You have been made aware of the needs of local humans by the nurses presently around you, so you also know of the needs for healing to those who are not mobile, but need the greatest of healing concentration, for their well being and life expectancy.

God Bless You... Amen

Chapter 10

Lister Hospital Day 8
24/05/08

Dr Ruth Kendall.

I come to oversee your condition as the Senior Earth Spirit Medic to make sure you are progressing in an even and constructive manner. Adjustments have been made to your form which are now in place and will begin to be activated, once the physical body has healed and returned to normal balance and animated quickness.

This is a time to consolidate the new energy within your body form and to give you time to receive the summer healing vibrations, when sunshine and natures bounty are at their highest.

Relish the time <u>now</u> - for you know that when momentum begins, it gathers force to take you along with it, and then there will be little time for personal pursuits.

26/05/08..........Left Hospital......

Liberation: to set free from the confines of your present situation.
The healing begins in earnest as you work towards physical normality. The etheric vehicles are now balanced and harmonized and are working to bring the physical form into unity, harmony and peace. You have much to assimilate as the experience has opened concepts and ideas for your consideration. The art of healing is extensive and takes many forms. It is the bringing together of like minded peoples who will work with you, to carry the healing work forward and outward into new areas of expertise.

In doing so the education begins, about the constructions of human form and the energy vehicles that have bearing upon the physical body.

A holistic approach is advocated as an ideal, but circumstances of physical life do not always allow for optimum circumstances to ensue, and compromises are always made, when we have to work with energy and vibrations that are immediately available. In time the other components can be allowed in, as the life circumstances change and move on.

That is why healing may take a little time, as each step of progress has to be consolidated upon the physical level. It is like a child using building blocks who wishes to create a construction in the right sequence, to show the correct colour code and match, for the structure as a whole.

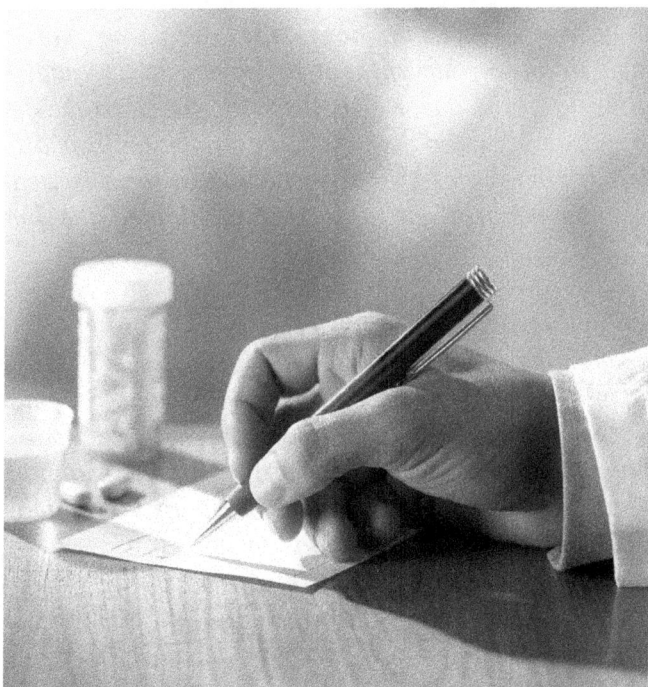

Prescription for Life

Chapter 11

Making that Connection
01/06/08

I had been given a C.D. entitled Tranquillity by my neighbour, to assist in my recovery from the recent major operation. The sounds of waves, music and bird song lifted my spirits to the sounds emitted, so that my inner voices became audible:-

The sound of waves, gently calm the frayed nerves of the emotions and mental vehicles, so that a more even tempo of the registration of the airwaves can be discerned.

As each wave ebbs and flows the breathing corresponds accordingly to the rhythm of the wave power. In the quiet you can hear the music of the oceans, as the wave force establishes itself upon the senses. Now the inner journey can begin. It is difficult to assemble the energy, for the physical unit of form is weak, after its life saving medical attention that eliminated the nugget of negative debris.

The inner soul awakens from its deep sleep to rejoin the living life of physical living. The new dawn of life activity begins with a gentle opening of the energy centres in unison to the sounds of the waves of the oceans and the bird song overhead. Bells are heard to summon the celestial influence as at the Sabbath it is appropriate to summon the spiritual forces, as they celebrate the symbolic day of rest to glory in Gods creativeness.

As the wave power becomes stronger, the power vibrates within your form, so you can feel the strength becoming a viable factor within your constitution.

The light of the Cosmic Christ shines upon you as you connect to the worlds of light and love. Your crusader waits to welcome you and take you within the confines of the banqueting hall where all the other masters and knights assemble.

*Here, groups are gathered in conversation and discussion, and it is to one of these groups you are directed. We are pleased that you have been able to journey here. Our conference is to discuss the viability of supplying your **Centre of Light** with additional energies to awaken those that call upon your services.*

We are actively encouraging all to wake up to the call of Gods awakening directive, so that all who hold within their hearts that recognition of conscious spiritual heritage, may become aware of their own divinity.

It is important that everyone who connects with the worlds of love and light are numbered and actively involved in the forward thrust of the present movement, to bring greater awareness and enlightenment to the mass of humans.

To recognise openly the spirit within, will bring that knowledge that you are not alone. You are a part of the great cosmic family which encompasses all within its form and frame, to manifest as the seen and unseen manifestations of creation.

All That Is.

In connecting with your spirit within, you make that connection with the Godhead which enables the communicative channels to connect with the many entities of spirit, who are available to guide and assist in the personal and collective life of the living present.

In doing so you become one of the awakened light workers who are gathering together to form an army upon the earth, of those people who understand the purpose and appreciate the necessity of working, to open the hearts and minds of others, to glory at the wonderment of the present life and age. You become a facilitator, a teacher, an instructor, a guide, a friend, a colleague, a server to God and Man. You become the link between the seen and unseen worlds which are drawing ever closer, so when they intermingle and produce windows of phenomenon, you will be able to explain and describe the significance of such events.

That which is different or unknown is always feared by those who do not as yet understand or accept new things as normal or natural. In this age of great change many things will need explanations, until the mass of humans can accept their changing world and embrace all that is. With understanding, acceptance becomes easier. Some will be quicker than others in the assimilation of new experiences and others will welcome change more readily than those who are set in their ways.

Be ever vigilant and resilient, for the world of man is fraught with unexpected obstacles, and there are those who love to trip up a fellow operator, in order to propel their own status upwards. We advise you to keep your feet firmly upon the ground and try to live a regulatory life, to bring an even tempo to the living life which will hold the high ground, when challenges are met.

Hold on to the light *and love within. Know this is your connection to us when outwardly the conditions are volatile. Hold the living flame within your hands and the healing light will flow through you to others. Hold the image of the flame within your minds eye and see the expanse of the light influence when in contrast with surrounding darkness.*

Hold the knowledge that you are never alone, your guardian guide walks with you. If you have any worries, hand them over to your guide and you will find that the weight and burden of cares are lifted from you, in such a way that the life events can be dealt with in an orderly and positive manner, and you will find that the weight carried, is only the amount you can manage.

Chapter 12

Testing the Connection
07/06/08

In the evening air, in the stillness of early evening, the only sounds around, are those of the birds making ready for their nights sojourn, and the insects hovering over the closing flowers within the confines of the garden boarders.

Cats silently parade the grass and banks and settle in quiet observation to judge any movement that occurs, as they bask in fulfilment and satisfaction in the aftermath, of consuming their evening meal. The sun is setting and casting its glow warmly over the landscape, as it descends into the horizon of the northern hemisphere.

The Crusader Knight stands on the sidelines waiting for all the distractions to abate, so that the stillness reigns within. Now he can step forward to communicate, as the human channel opens for receptivity:

This particular receptive channel has only recently re-opened due to the necessary priority of the physical demands upon the vehicle of the form, to whom the channel belongs.

In the recuperative time when healing rays have begun to filter through to the physical, to have their effect in re-vitalising the areas that have recently been injured, due to the removal of a concentrated nugget of negativity, which amalgamated all the offending material within the form body, so that it could be removed and eliminated, to leave a cleaner vehicle for us to use.

It is to be said that this form body of the one who houses the channel of communication, is one that is being monitored for future work and deliveries of knowledge and information, which can and will have great impact upon the humans of connectivity, to aid in the development and understanding of the masses in future times. To this end we are testing the mechanism of communication as you would expect to test any new equipment which is a communicative system or innovation.

To hear spirit you must be still and quiet. Once the correct frequency is found, then this communicative airway can be switched on, at times when the mind can consciously attune.

It is beneficial if the timing of communications can be regulated, as this sets up an appointment time, when personnel on both sides of the communicating stream, are placed for positive broadcast and reception. It is like switching on the news station at set times, for morning and evening, to become a regular occurrence of daily activity.

Once this regularity has become established, the free flow of information can be readily transmitted, as a programme of timely knowledge can be systematically imparted. The initial communication is one of appreciation and acknowledgement that the greater awareness of natural things and nature is registering more acutely.

At present the heavy foliage around your habitat brings a heavy coating of deep green, to aid in the balance and harmony of your emotional and mental vehicles. The colours of the flowers within your garden have been registered as mauve & purple, white and gold. The white flowers always accompany the coloured varieties, as if to stamp the creators signature upon the array of manifestation. The coloured fruits becoming ripe, give credence to the fact that the abundance of natures hoard is fruitful and fulfilling the cycle of its life force.

All is in order.
All is as it should be.
All is balanced.
All is harmonious.

The equilibrium is sought and maintained.
Enjoy this peace time.
BE
For as you come to the realisation of your stillness and being, you become aware of the connection of your spirit to the unseen, and connect with the etheric dimensions. You can see with your inner eyes as the blue white light streaks across the two connection points, to unite the stream of energy now connected, one with the other.

The Crusader and Knights welcome you to the banqueting hall for once again you have journeyed to our meeting place. We gather in groups for discussions and debate, as you would expect elders to deliberate. You are part of the team which decides on the manner of how knowledge can be imparted to the students upon earth.

As an earth light-worker, it is people like you who are asked to deliver information, and the manner it is delivered or imparted carries great responsibility. If the delivery is sympathetically administered to the various key workers, the benefits will be seen as a wide distribution. If the opposite occurs, the vital or needed information will die an immediate death. It is important that in all communications between spirit and man, the highest of motives and standards are sought, to insure the integrity of all participants and receivers alike.

When the highest of ideals is activated in all that is carried out within the communicating network, then the quality cannot be in questioned and the source no longer dismissed as fanciful, but revered as valuable and above reproach.

Know that your contribution is noted and welcomed. We again endorse your efforts to the cause of enlightenment.

God Bless You.

Chapter 13

Tuesday 10/06/08
The Healing and the Connection
Hitchin Church Service 7.30pm

It was Tuesday 10th June 2008. I was feeling particularly low in energy and vulnerable and in need of healing. The day before I had attended another centre for healing but no healers were operating that day, due to holidays and a week of Congress which many were attending.

I had advocated healing to patients while in hospital and given details of where healing was available in the local area of North Hertfordshire for each day of the week. It suddenly occurred to me that I should avail myself of the healing available, as I was as much in need as anyone else.

Hence, I called upon people I know, and was duly transported to the evening service for healing. Upon my arrival I found a friendly face of old, a fellow student of mediumship and a healer that I had not seen for some time, so a catch up chat ensued.

I asked my friend to provide healing and no sooner had hands been laid upon my shoulders, when I saw clairvoyantly an hour glass. This indicated to me, that healing was being passed from the spirit world to the earth world, as the grains of sand gently flowed from top to bottom.

I then became aware of a black African man with a shaven head, who wore large earrings of bone. Around his neck and shoulders he sported a wide collar of coloured beads, decorated discs, animal teeth and bone fragments. This was an African Witch Doctor with big brown eyes that looked straight at me, face to face, as if he was only a few feet away.

I next saw him sitting cross legged upon a high hill, looking over the landscape and watching the clouds as they passed overhead.

My viewpoint joined him and I began to realise that the clouds were gathering speed and the landscape disappeared, as I was registering the sensation of clouds all around me rushing past. I felt that time was speeding up to transport me to another place.

As the speed slowed, I became aware of the landscape once again. I was nearing a sea shore, a small bay enclosed by cliffs. Upon the shore and set a little distance back, but in full view of the sea and sand, was a glass bubble or biosphere.

This was the healing place to which I was directed. How I knew this, I do not know. The place was very tranquil and all seemed balanced and in harmony with the surrounding coastline, sea rhythm and shore.

Within this glass dome I could see the sea, gently ebbing and flowing upon the beach. This set up and maintained the rhythm, which set the mind and emotions at peace. All was quiet, except for the natural sounds gently forming a background tempo.

I was directed to a healing pod which housed a couch and was covered with a transparent lid. Within this pod I underwent a light therapy, where white light was radiated into my body, to saturate each organ and cell and to re-vitalise those parts which had recently been subjected to physical trauma and required adjustment and healing. I felt highly charged and invigorated, and my mind was once again clear. After a short space of time, I was duly directed back to the here and now within the healing circle.

I was next shown a number of letters posted through a letterbox that landed on the inside doormat. Amongst this post were coloured envelopes, which indicated to me that they were birthday cards or get well cards.

This was confirmation to me that spirit recognised my recent birthday which coincided with the many get-well cards I had received for my recuperation.

I suddenly realised I had made the connection which I had sought, and tested out the communicative pathway, which took me to another dimension for healing. I had also made that connection with the guides who work with me, to provide clairvoyant images when relaying information and knowledge.

I was back in business as a working medium.
I smiled with satisfaction and thankfulness.
I slept well that night and had pleasant dreams.

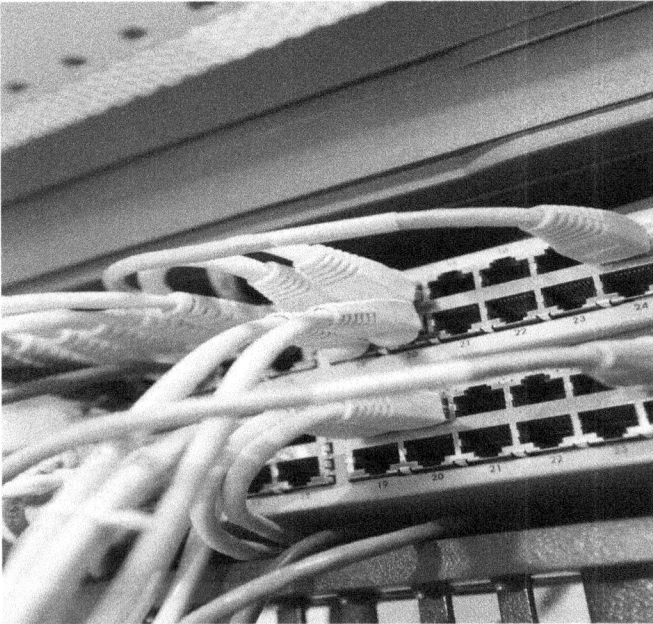

Connections

Chapter 14

Friday 13th June 2008
The Energy Healing Centre
Letchworth Library.

After attending the Doctors surgery to have my wound dressed and finding I had another infection brewing, I went home to start the course of anti-biotic treatment prescribed and given.

I felt somewhat low in spirits as I had received some very good healing a few days earlier and felt I was definitely on the mend, so I wondered how I had regressed so quickly. It occurred to me later that sometimes you have to take a step backwards in order to take two steps forward. This I believe was one of those occasions.

I asked my neighbour for a lift to the Energy Healing Centre which operated on a Friday afternoon, where I hoped to receive a Reiki session. Lynda as a friend and the Reiki therapist had visited me in hospital twice, so I felt I should support her as best I could. I thought I would take along my Tarot Cards, just in case they were needed for a reading, as the thought had crossed my mind. I was being optimistic as I hadn't really given a personal reading since my hospitalisation and certainly wasn't in the best of health or fitness when it came to my physical body.

I arrived just after 4pm to find that Lynda was on her own and with only one patient booked for a 4.30pm slot. I was fortunate to be able to receive healing straight away. The moment I laid upon the healing table and had closed my eyes, I saw clairvoyantly, my Nun Guide filing her finger nails in a nonchalant manner. This perplexed me for a moment as her attitude seemed to be one of 'well, we are waiting'.

Nothing immediately came to mind as to why I was being shown this rather astounding vision. As soon as the healing began, my

Nun got to work by distributing summer flowers all around me, to make up an outer body line. Suddenly the sun within my visionary eye shone upon me, and was captured by these flowers, forming a circumference.

This set up an energy force field which covered me as in a dome and was anchored by all the flowers around me, providing the border. This was the healing capsule reconstructed in a different location but achieving the same healing quality and force I had received a few days before, while receiving healing at another spiritual healing centre.

After my Reiki healing session the next appointment arrived, so I helped out with this healing session and found my hands heating up and tingling as of old. I also picked up the emotional turmoil of this patient and then went on to give a reading to this lady. With the help of those in spirit I was able to give an inspired session of counselling, that was very well received as it was exactly what this lady needed.

At 5.30pm when I had intended to leave, another person also wanted a reading, so I again I found myself engaged in sorting out another persons life and their relationship problems. At the end of the afternoon, I understood my Nuns attitude: she had been waiting for me to start work. I thanked her for the healing given and also for the opportunity to work and test the communicative channel.

Lynda had stated earlier, that she was behind with the bills and hadn't paid the rent or advertising last week, as no one had turned up. We made up for the loss of the previous week by the takings received that afternoon, so Lynda was able to restore the balance to this working healing centre, which offers a worthwhile service as a drop in centre.

What occurred is an example in physical reality of the working out of trust in spirit. If your trust is in spirit both sides of the veil, you will always be re-reimbursed for energy given out and services rendered. All will be restored to balance.

So have faith in your beliefs and ask those in spirit for assistance when required. Know that spirit will never let you down as this has been proved, time and time again.

Learn from examples and reap the rewards to see your services bear results............. Blessing to All.

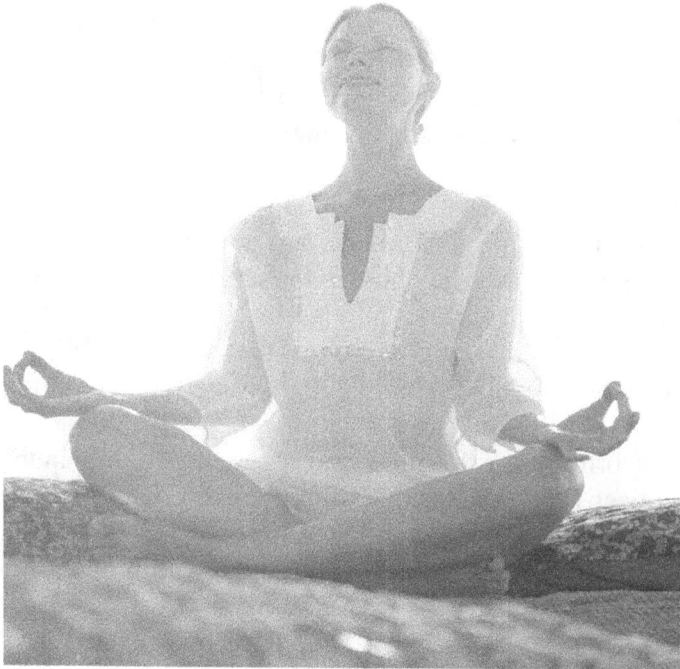

Attunement

Chapter 15

Summer Solstice
21/06/08

The year of consolidation has reached its half way point and you may observe that what has manifested upon the physical plane has been one of drastic sorting and shifting between the poles of duality.

Much has been crystallised to become visible and therefore can, and has in some cases, been dealt with by elimination of the negativity, to allow that which is positive or natural to be freed from any constraints. This process has and will allow those who have suffered negative health, personal relationships, adverse living or financial blows, to progress forward in their spiritual or natural understanding, which encompasses the higher values of life and living. A new way forward is postulated to engage the interests of those who need to change.

Many light workers are awakening to the new energy patterns pervading the Earth. The effects are to purify those individuals who potentially have the abilities for service to their brothers and sisters. The wake up call may seem harsh, but is effective, as humans require a strong stimulus, that is powerful enough to overshadow or colour all other things within the living life.

A crisis brings re-evaluation and assessment, both individually and collectively. This is the turning point within the year of consolidation, following the year of change, where so many are facing a crisis of sorts, to bring changes within and without. In consolidating all that is good, beautiful and true, it may mean the elimination or discarding of those things within life and living that cause disharmony.

Past and accumulative conditions lodged within forms are being eliminated, so health and welfare for some, becomes a prime consideration for present attention. In others a financial crisis looms to herald in changes within their lifestyle, which may have been previously highlighted, but not yet activated and brought into the present reality, which by necessity is now required.

Others, of which there appears to be many, include the various changes and alterations within relationships. Personal, Corporate, Friendship links are all changing, as many are affected by the current energies relayed to earth, the effects of which bring about an examination of values. This call to examine enables many humans to once again look towards their spiritual heritage, and their connection to the Great Creator, from an individual viewpoint and not from any collective indoctrination.

Crisis in all departments of living and life brings soul searching to the masses. It is no longer enough to accept what man has broadcast as a living philosophy, as the affects can be seen crumbling all around you like a pack of cards falling to the ground. What has been built on shifting sands will ultimately dissolve and disappear. In present times, the quickening of souls by the effects of the finer energies transmitted to earth, is seen in human consciousness, as confirmed by the many who are questioning the circumstances of their existence.

In all areas of life, the organisations of old and new are also re-examining their mode of operandi. It seems that a return to basics can bring a new enlightenment, as old values are re-examined and new ideas sifted for added value. This way a more solid foundation can be built, upon which to base understanding, ideology and philosophy, for the physical life experience.

Many humans have already made inroads to change the existing working organisations that abound within societies. Some have gone overboard and are following a route of change for changes sake. Others lag behind in unstable regimes.

Because of the widespread differences found upon the physical earth, it is required that everyone change in some way, so all the fractions of society in all areas and nations, can move towards an overall level and balance, in order to bring about a synthesis of the species. Much work towards good relations between all humans is ongoing by those who see the creators plan clearly. No nation or sets of people can exist in isolation. No one nation can have ultimate power over others. Co-operation is the key and a way found through the mass of differences.

Hearts should be opened and examples of compassion displayed. Goodness is not weakness, when happiness and wellbeing is of paramount importance. If you show by example, many will be enamoured of your example and voluntarily wish to emulate the pattern or example displayed. This way your influence will be greater than any imposition of human will, for all that is positively applied will be beneficial, and all that which is imposed becomes short lived.

Consolidate all that you know to be right, beneficial, good and true. Keep all things as simple as you can, for simple things can be understood by everyone. Love your neighbour as best you can and show by example within your own personal life, how co-operation can benefit those around you. By adopting these principles and values you will find a greater peace within your own soul, as you realise that you have done all you can to bring peace and harmony to the circle of influence you serve. Multiply this by all humans and soon the world could be transformed. The light of reason and love spreads far and wide once the initial spark has ignited.

Those in spirit are waiting for your action, so they too can play their part in the forward revolving of momentum. The light of illumination will be given to those who start the changes within their own lives, so that the light of spirit can shine through the visages of human faces, to consolidate the plan and direction of the coming age.

Know that the light workers of the present age which are upon your earth world are attracting others to unite. Through the light organisations which encompass healing, teaching, spirituality and personal development and understanding, the light of each soul increases.

Consolidate your knowing, by joining groups who wish to further their knowledge and expertise in the many fields of human service, which combine with Gods service to humanity. By joining with the forward thrust of endeavour, you will find a purpose growing within you, to transform all about you into goodness and beauty. Look at nature in your own garden. See the beauty manifesting at summer solstice, when the bounty of flowers are decorating the borders of many gardens, public places and displays in garden centres and homes. Notice the variety of colours that abound at this time for all the colours are being shown to attract the insects and smaller creatures.

Remember one kingdom inter-relates to another, both above and below, so all kingdoms manifested in the physical world of earth and joining as one, become dependant upon each other. The flowering and the fruitfulness of summer's bounty precedes the harvest, so look for the developments of goodness, which become generated from the more purified forms and endeavours of human activity.

Look to the ideology adopted which is more simple and pure in concept.

Look into your hearts to see the truth in all things and know that the simple seed of understanding is within all, from which to grow and flower to perfection.......Amen.

Chapter 16

Summers Energy.
30/06/08

There are many students of the mystic arts who have made great strides upon the spiritual pathway by their dedication and services upon the earth, to aid and better the conditions of humankind.

Many have grown in spiritual understanding and now face a crisis within their own lives, because of the physical and material circumstances around them, which are appearing contradictory to all they would desire. The face of change is upon the landscape, as the soul battles to understand the relevance of the two opposing dimensions, and somehow it has to reconcile the two, in order that he or she may move forward in unity, with both aspects of their nature and understanding in equal balance.

This is a difficult time for any soul which is facing great challenges, brought about by the quickening of the etheric vehicles, in response to the cosmic or spiritual stimuli presently relayed from the greater universe. At varying times in a human life cycle the individual may be faced by what they describe as a crossroads, where a decision made or a direction taken today, will have far reaching effects upon the morrow. This is were the spiritual self and the physical self, stand face to face, and the lower and higher self's are matched against each other.

The lower self will not give up with out resistance, so the individual has to suffer the agonies of mental and emotional turmoil, before the lower self will resign itself to the command of its higher counterpart, which will then lead the life experience into new areas for self discovery upon the path of growth. Many times the progress of a soul has to face this type of stand, where the travel is halted for examination and understanding. The struggle may manifest as an injury or illness or even a relationship change, which the individual must resolve and overcome in order to move forward.

This involves the mental and emotional aspects of the living human to concentrate upon the physical, in order to activate the self healing properties into action, and to channel the healing energies abounding to the receptive body parts of the physical form, and to those aspects that effect mental or emotional relationships. By invocation and concentration of directed positive thoughts and actions, it is possible to make the necessary changes to bring in line, the balancing of the lesser vehicles of human makeup, to align with the spiritual growth that has been achieved.

Finding the keys to bring this balancing and harmonizing about is not easy, as every aspect of life and living needs re-examining. Some may need to go back in time and deal with issues as yet unresolved. Often physical ailments can manifest in later life by events of childhood or youth, where issues covered up, may reveal hidden debris, which requires clearing and elimination.

This is where a good housekeeping clearance is needed. At summer time the days are bright and sunny, so for practical purposes of cleaning and clearing out, the climate is right for such activities to take place. If everyone took upon themselves the spring cleaning of the physical and then the summer shine of the emotions and mindsets, a harvest of renewal would surely unfold.

So if you have problems appearing in earthly life for which the answers are not apparent, look into your past, re-examine the areas of your present life to see where changes and clearance would be beneficial. For those who are presently experiencing a crisis manifestation in the living life, know that this event represents a challenge and opportunity for future growth and development. It may not seem relevant to you, when you are facing calamities of sorts, but all things are brought about by actions present and past.

What you have sown in the past has a way of manifesting in the present, and this applies to both the good and not so good. Life is to be lived and it is a very cleaver human who understands that living the material life, is the means to meet the challenges of what life presents. Large and small are the lessons given for each and every one. Some souls may seem to have a lack lustre life while others seemed to have been born under a lucky star. It is the karma of your chosen life, the blueprint of your present lifespan.

Be like a willow and bend with the wind. Allow the life circumstances to flow around you but not touch you. Become like an oasis within the desert. Become like a calm spot within a storm. Become a light shinning within the darkness, while all around panic and make no headway, while you have stopped to align you energies with the higher vibrations of love and light to move steadily forward under divine guidance.

This action will bring you clarity of sight and reveal a pathway through the presented turmoil. When you have travelled a little further along the pathway of life, the unveiling of truths is revealed. As each snippet of knowledge becomes realised within your consciousness, then you will find that the crossroads of yesterday was but a start of a new phase of learning, to bring you into the realisation of greater truths.

Life is for learning by experience and observation. If we do not take notice by observation or historic information given to us, we find ourselves experiencing circumstances outside of our imaginations. It is at summers high when energies are at an apex. This brings an opportunity to access these high energies for human use.

Let the summer sun bring light and warmth to all the adverse circumstances that presently manifest in earthly lives, so that the mindsets and emotional vehicles of each and every one can experience the upliftment of natures sunshine, and bring about the harvest of bounty which evolves from this high time of year.

Know that the seasons revolve according to the planets own cosmic cycles, which impinge their influence upon the planetary life and all that inhabits its inner and outer boundaries.

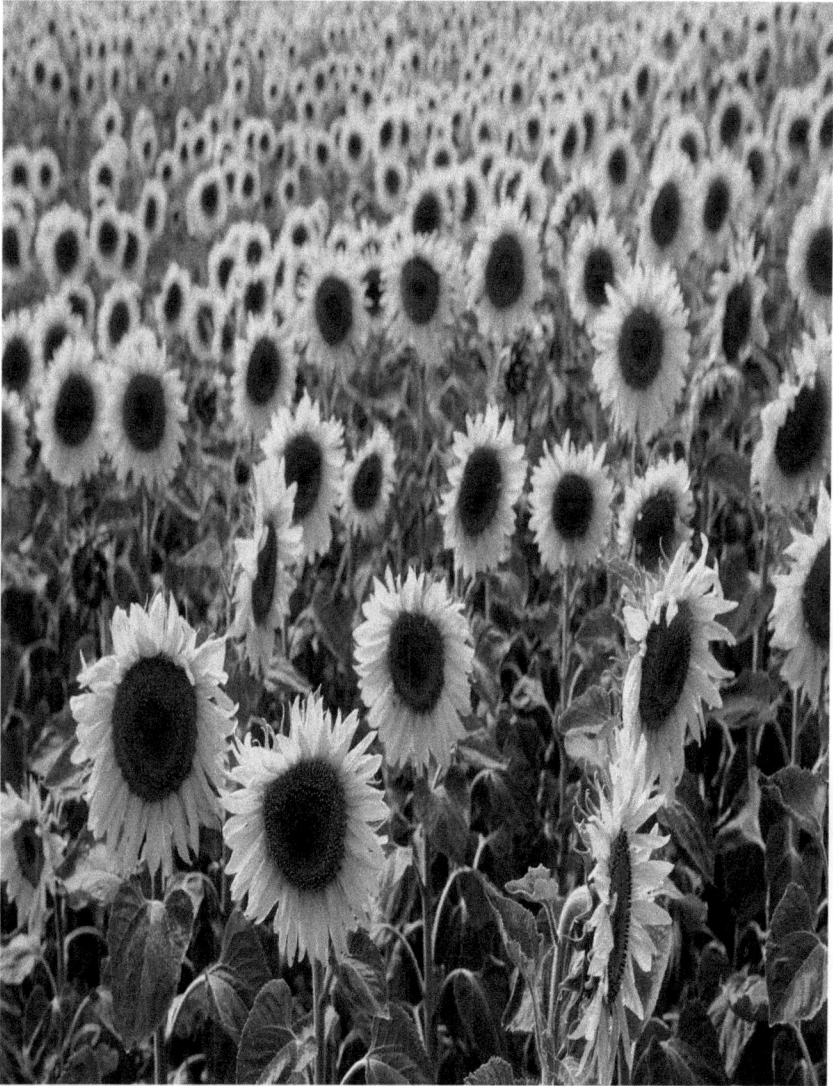

Summers Glory

Chapter 17

Waterfall of Light
30/06/08

I sat in the midst of a circle of healers while healing energy was directed to me from all around. I became aware of this surge of energy as a flame, lightening up and expanding its light far and wide. The colour changed from warm red to light purple and an expansion of consciousness was registered.

I felt my inner self rise up out of the confines of my physical form to take on a Buddha silhouette. As it did so, my awareness shifted in unison with my higher vehicle, and I stood as the Buddhic principal by the side of a welcoming Master, who stood patiently waiting for me. This master looked like the Christ and for some reason this did not surprise me at all.

As I took my place beside the Master I registered the surroundings of cool blue and white, and thought that this was the place for healing. I detected some activity of healing being carried out, as I looked at the walls of the light corridor and saw scenes and images.

As the thought entered my mind that this was a healing area, we began to travel and I was manoeuvred through the corridors of the light and light vortexes, to bring me to a place of tranquillity, where a stream of light cascaded as a waterfall into the stream below.

At the waters edge and built onto the right hand side of a rocky cliff face, which enclosed this place on either side, was a palace building of some beauty. Resembling an Arabian palace with balconies and round turrets in cream and gold, there was one large balcony overhanging the stream, which looked like it was within touching distance of the waterfall itself.

Somehow I landed upon this balcony and was ushered through the French doors, into a large cool room with high ceilings and plenty of light. Here a mother lady was sitting crossed legged upon a large emerald green cushion.

This mother lady was richly dressed as an Indian wearing a sari and I felt she was a mixture of Indian with Buddhic origins. She was busy teaching the children about her, who were also sitting cross legged in a semi-circle.

There were eight children in all, and I stood behind them watching what was going on and wondering what it all meant. The children were dressed in rich clothes which somehow depicted their origin. There were five boys and three girls of ages ranging between five and eleven years of age in human terms.

There was a boy about ten years of age who was white skinned with blue eyes and had bright golden hair. He had an angelic face which glowed. His colouring stood out from the other children who were all darker in comparison. There was a small Red Indian girl about five years old who hung onto his tunic, and looked up to him, mesmerised by his countenance.

I noticed another boy about seven who was oriental and another girl who I definitely took to be Chinese. The third girl was olive skinned with long curly hair, who reminded me of a gypsy child with dark haunting eyes with hidden depths. The other boys I identified as one black African, one Arab and one Indian who was the eldest and wore a turban.

The mother lady was showing the children how to use light energy balls in a controlled and balanced manner, and to use thoughts to create and balance these light balls held above each hand, so they could be carried to the balcony.

The eldest boy was asked to provide a demonstration. He balanced a light ball in his hand very steadily and kept it levitated about six inches above the palm. He threw it or more correctly he released it, into the area above the stream.

I expected it to drop and form part of the stream below, but this did not happen. Instead the energy light ball began to spin and create a spiral vortex of energy within the atmosphere above the stream, to suddenly disappear into another dimension. I seemed to know this automatically.

As my attention looked up from this happening, I realised I could see what can only be described as a conveyor belt emerging from the left hand side of the waterfall and passing through the centre of it. Upon the conveyor belt were outlines of human forms which I registered as shapes of souls, who had been brought here for healing and purifying.

As the souls passed through the light waterfall, they were immersed in this energy light which acts as fire-light to purify, and heals like water, to unify and balance the being, into renewed wholeness.

The conveyor belt moved slowly through the waterfall of light to emerge into the sunshine of the atmosphere. This is where the soul forms receive their sparkle, as you would expect, if they were a crystal gem receiving a shine when washed, cleaned and polished.

The other children came to the balcony with their light orbs shining above their hands and I witnessed each one, throw their light energy ball to one of the souls upon the conveyor belt, who were returning to their own time and dimension.

This I knew, was to give a newly configured soul, a great gift of the power of healing and wisdom, so they may take to their own dimension in time and space, this clarity of knowing, and the ability of transmitting this Christ energy of love.

Coming directly from the wisdom of the ages, this great healing power of the universe is the pure essence of sublime love, emanating from our Great and loving Creator.

The children returned to the lady mother and were praised for their efforts, and the excellence and accuracy of their endeavours. Suddenly a door opened at the far end of the room and a male father figure stepped into the room.

He was dressed in the Indian clothes of a Rajah and exuded a great presence. The children all stood up and with excitement ran to greet him.

I saw this father figure, open his arms and send out his love to the children and witnessed an outflow ripple of such magnitude, which showed the energy encircling all the children within its circumference.

I can only describe this event as viewing a sizable ripple that takes place in water, when an object is immersed in its still state, causing a ripple of movement of some volume in relation to the size of the original energy displacement and movement.

I knew, with all that I had witnessed at this place, that this was a healing station where youngsters in this realm, learned the arts of wielding energies for balancing and harmonising forms and structures of many dimensions, within the gambit of the universal spheres, which this healing station serves.

I became aware that I had been guided to this place so that I could visit here myself in times of need, for the purpose of healing, since at this time I am undergoing a programme of in depth healing and purification of the inner being as well as the fortification of the physical body.

I had been told by my guides a little time ago, that in my recuperative time while physical healing takes place, those who work with me would provide new knowledge and information, upon which I should write.

I believe this experience is one of these lessons, providing insight into what occurs in other dimensions, which can affect our own existence, when invocations of need are met with positive results.

Since my own health has been highlighted, the healing of others has become of paramount importance to me. In particular, it is those aspects relating to the practical applications of healing, in its various and many forms.

This is why the knowledge on healing, affecting the etheric vehicles is required, so that all the vehicles or levels that make up the whole human body form can be attended to, in the correct manner.

Many of the problems now manifesting upon the physical form arise as a result of some irregularity or blockage upon one of the unseen levels.

When the new age medic is called to assess the problem of one soul in particular, he must view the soul in a unified manner in order to treat the true cause and not just the physical effect.

If by the use of meditation and the ability of healing sessions to release our inner being to be healed in their own dimension, we can begin to formulate a new and revolutionary way to redress any unbalance, and bring health and happiness back to those who have momentarily lost their way.

I returned to my place in the earthly circle of healing, full of white light and upliftment.

I thank all who sent me this healing energy, from both the seen and unseen dimensions, and the lesson and knowledge imparted.

Chapter 18

Garden of Colour Healing.
01/07/08

The Healers of All Souls is a spiritual healing group which meets on Wednesday afternoons at Letchworth Garden City.

This was the seventh week after my major operation and everyone commented on how well I was looking. My healing this afternoon took me straight away to a country meadow.

I became a young girl skipping and dancing in the meadow dressed in a summer frock, and with a garland of flowers around my head. This I registered as hands were placed upon my brow. I had two people acting the healers, one at the front and the other at my back.

The summer suns heat was felt by the hands upon my front and the coolness of running water was felt from the hands upon my back. The summer sun brought me into a garden of flowers. It seemed as if all the flowers and plants were of a gigantic size and I was but the size of an insect.

A drop of moisture dripped from a yellow bell, which looked like a bluebell coloured yellow, yet it was gigantic in comparison. The drop of moisture was like an instant shower, that covered me fully and momentarily, I felt drenched with the shock of this occurrence. Like a dog shakes its coat to rid itself of water, I shook my head in like manner, to eliminate the excess moisture.

This felt rejuvenating. I felt rejuvenated as I registered this imagery which was evoked from the healing energy given. I found myself walking in a golden meadow amongst the ripe corn. A feeling of freeness became my senses as I strolled carefree along the meadow. The summers sun was again felt in full force, as the picture of me drying out, was pleasantly invigorating, as I returned to normal consciousness.

The impression of the enlarged flowers and the meadow I had encountered during my healing session remained with me for some hours, so I linked again to this imagery, to see if there was anything I had missed and I asked my guide to provide insight. I realised immediately that I was again as a young girl moving freely about, without cares or worries of any kind.

This I understood was a lesson to me to remember that at a young age, the troubles of life were not evident and the appreciation of nature was something that was encountered with pure joy and glee. I was reminded, not to let earthly problems effect me in any major way, as this over time, will result in diseasements. Adopting a viewpoint that is pure and unaffected by others, in thought or deed is advocated. Accordingly, this can manifest to become a wonderful encounter of spirits, between the nature sprites and humans.

Natures elementals are the builders of form and all things that grow and have their existence during the seasons of natural occurrence, is the product of the creative measure of those unseen, who live to make physical manifestations, the natural phenomenon, which we as humans take so much for granted.

The cycle of natures seasons and life cycles of vegetation are lessons for humans to note, so they may understand the relevance within their own life. For me, it is the regeneration of form into a new cycle of living as I enter my Indian summertime of glory. To re-create the conditions of when young can be attained in vibration terms, as the renewal of energies take place. Within the human physical body, the life blood of each form, regenerates and changes its total volume every quarter.

This is the mirror image of the seasons taking place within our own form, without us necessarily knowing or feeling any effect, other than registering the effects of the outward climate of our environment. To consciously purify our form we must undertake a three monthly detoxification regime, whereby we begin to change the input of food and liquids, to consume more pure and natural forms containing the higher concentration of life energy known a Chi or Qi or Ki.

It is this life energy which flows through each living thing, which aids to strengthen and emerge as a great flow of vitality. This manifests as vigour and wellbeing, together with mental alertness of clarity, which translates as clear vision and knowing. During this process to restore the balance of strength within the physical form, the diseasements of yesterday are eased and the present form registers, as more harmonious and balanced, in all ways concerning its energy frequencies.

Often the diseased problem has vanished altogether as the positive vibrations have transformed the negative atoms into waste, which have been eliminated from the form by natural means. If some past diseasments have been major, then a substantial reduction in size and volume of the problem will occur. Further positive healing with colour vibrations to specific areas of the form, can then be administered, and with rest and loving care, a person may return to normal life and living. Not all cases of disease can be cured, for the karma of the individual has bearing upon the form. All however, can be helped and assisted in terms of wellbeing and upliftment.

To those whose diseasments must be endured, it is a case of living with a disability and rising above the effects, which this infirmity may bring. Attitude has a positive effect upon the healing of any form, as the thoughts of the being are able to receive or block the inflow of healing vibrations, as they enter into and are absorbed by the physical cell construction of the being.

It may be particularly important at this time to ground the physical form by indorsing all things relating to the earthly life and living. This may include reinforcing relationships and contacts, undertaking physical activities conducive to welfare and fitness.

The karma of any individual will determine the life gambit of the form, so some are surprised when healing seemingly does not work as the patient dies. It may be the case that the healing has indeed worked most effectively, to allow the release of the spirit from the bodily form.

That particular form may not have been robust enough to undertake and carry further the work set, for the forward programme of the soul, of which this one form personality is but a part. It is particularly a sensitive time when one of our loved ones is faced with a seemingly negative prognosis. In these cases we can only project the positive outcome of the fulfilment of life in a positive and balanced manner.

If the balancing of the scales is tipped to further the physical living, a time for recuperation and rejuvenation may ensue. The focus of life will have changed to take it in a new direction, so that new goals may be fulfilled.

If the scales are tipped towards the heavens and the return of the soul indicated, departing souls may resign themselves to contemplating and contacting the levels of love and light, so that the transition of form may be accomplished in peace and harmony. Love heals and will bridge the channels of all those connected by love, feeling and sensing.

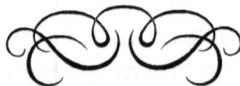

Chapter 19

I was considering a weeks training course at The Arthur Findlay College, Stansted, UK. This would be my convalescent treat so I could test the mechanism of spirit communication for public demonstration purposes.

After this healing meditation communication, I rang up the college to find that there was only one vacancy left for the 26th July 2008. I booked it. This will be my mental physiotherapy. I recently read that if it pleases the mind, then it will be good for the body.

The Address.

Tuesday 15th July 2008 Hitchin Church Healing Service.

It was quiet when I arrived at the church, just before the majority of people arrived, so I was able to sit in the silence in contemplation. The music was particularly tranquil as healers and those who had come to receive healing arranged themselves, sitting on the chairs that had been placed in a circle.

I had two people administering healing to me and I was straight away aware of a Red Indian prancing around me and extracting shafts of white stuffing from my form and grumbling at the amount of negative debris I had accumulated in just a week.

I then became aware of my Nun Guide who took me to a crowded room where I/she stood to give an inspired talk to those assembled. I was urged to talk to the crowd and relay my nuns words. It was a training week for mediums who had gathered together for instructions. I became the instrument of delivery while my Nun Guide inspired my spoken words.

Greetings to all those who have travelled far, to join with their colleagues at this meeting house. You shine your faces to me, with excitement and in anticipation of what might transpire.

You have all assembled with the expectation of a week of hard work in fine-tuning your channels of connectivity and re-enforcing those abilities and gifts by practising your teaching skills for the many students that will come your way.

We are all preparing at this time, for the influx of new entrants into the mystical arts. This is because the many young people who are now maturing into adulthood, are now recognising that the impulses, sensing and phenomenon experienced in childhood, have a real meaning and purpose, and the urgency of the need to know and connect to the sources of this phenomenon is of an urgency that is now gathering force to some great degree.

Many young humans are frustrated at the lack of knowledge around them and they are compelled to seek others of like mind, so that they may unite and exchange experiences. It is important to such humans, that your endeavours here at this time are successful, for they will be relying upon all of you, to provide the missing information they seek.

Many young humans are confused. They seek the connection to spirit which you can provide and the training and expertise necessary, to provide a discipline to work with, which is needed if the skills of today are to be handed to the next generation of active spirit channels. This is particularly important as the calibre of tomorrows medium, will need to be much greater than some at present in operation.

This is because the finer energies are relayed in a slightly different manner and the reception of these vibrations, are such, that the sensitive human working medium, needs to fine-tine their receptive mechanism. This is necessary to accommodate the wider scale of vibrational notes that are brought forth from the universal spheres, to enhance the wider colour and sound spectrums.

Since all levels have correspondences, the sensitive channel of tomorrow will need to be even more sensitive, or of a greater flexibility, in order to play all the octaves of an enlarged scale. To explain further, it is required that you understand the impact of the present changes taking place upon your world existence.

The ascension process will bring about an age where the finer energies will be more apparent than ever before. Ordinary humans will be able to demonstrate a certain level of awareness by showing their natural physic abilities in their natural everyday life activities. This will provide a basis or spring board for those who want to connect to spirit. This desire may be held, but not all gifted psychics have the discipline or ethics, to develop a channel of receptivity to the higher realms.

As many channels of broadcast become available for receptivity, only those who have the moral integrity should be encouraged to develop a channel to contact the higher realms, in order to receive communications from Light Beings, Angels and Ascended Masters. There will be a growing number of psychics who are attracted to the Earth Divas and will be connected to the earthly vibrations. This will be needed, as it will provide information and feedback that is required, if the changes within Mother Earth are to be understood.

It is to the calibre of the human individual that this training session is directed, for if spirit guides can instil the need for the best possible receptor to house the perfected mechanisms for high vibrational communications, then the expertise overall within the mediumistic fraternity will be enhanced. This will encourage others to work to a high level of attainment, and this will require sacrifice and training of all those involved.

You have a saying: 'there is no gain without pain'. In any attainment of worth there requires much dedication and service in the pursuit of the goal. Rest assured, the rewards for becoming an excellent communicator, who can demonstrate a clear and uncluttered channel for spirit communication, is a goal worth attaining.

There is so much of wonder that spirit can bring to human incarnates, with the wonderful messages from loved ones which are treasures indeed. It is only when you have lost a dear one that you can truly appreciate the significance of hearing from them again.

The healing, the upliftment, the glory of the connection cannot be stressed enough. Know that your time here this week is just the start of much work to come. Remember love is the working currency. I will speak again shortly. Thank-you for listening.

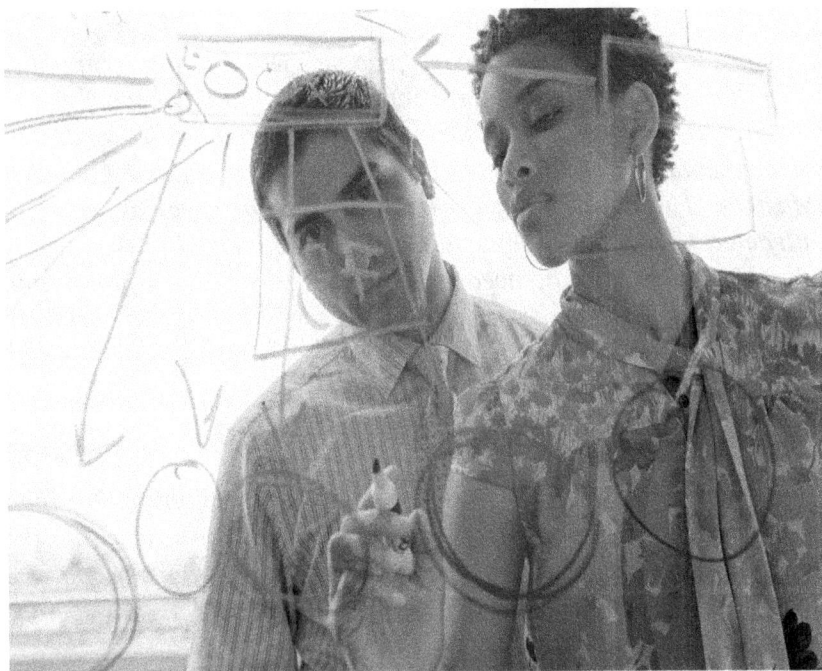

Learning

Chapter 20

Healing Service,
Hitchin Church
22/07/08

Sitting in a circle listening to music was the order of the healing service that evening. I went to Steve for my hands on healing, which placed me facing the church altar. Steve is training to be a trance healer and the year before, he had been one of my students in a development class for mental mediumship. As soon as the healing energy started to flow, I closed my eyes to find myself seeing clairvoyantly, with my head bent:

I was sitting with my head bowed in a state of utter despair. It was as if I had placed myself before God in Gods house as a last resort, as my emotional and mental self had reached rock bottom and I was bereft.

I had come for healing that evening as I had been overdoing things and had put my back out, so I was having difficulty with my walking and my hip joints were stiff. This had made me a little tired and low in spirits but nothing of major importance, as this healing exercise was part of my weekly ongoing therapy after my operation now some nine weeks ago.

I could not get over this feeling of overwhelming despair and desolation that was around me. I suddenly felt a pull upon my senses to raise my head and look at the altar. I registered a large cross upon the altar. My viewpoint rose from the bottom of the cross and followed upwards to the top in a straight line.

As I followed this line of vision, my view opened to show the heavens and it was as if the face of Christ was displayed before me. As I looked at this apparition, my sense of despair vanished and I was filled with hope and joy of knowing without doubt, that all was well. **My life was well as I had placed my trust in the almighty and my call had been ANSWERED.**

The scene faded to be replaced by faces of my guides and helpers, all showing their faces as if in confirmation. A Red Indian face was very strong in features and a presence seemed to say to me **'You have been told and now you know'.** *This was referring to my faith and belief in the spiritual understanding of our eternal existence and of miracles. My Nun showed her face and she smiled as if to say,* **'There, there, my child, you are not alone and your trust is well placed'.** *Tears of tension release fell down my face, as the light filled my being, as I was merged with the light energy of healing.*

My consciousness returned to the healing circle and I found my eyes moist and my body pleasantly tired but at peace. By the time I had returned home, I had this feeling that there was more to this experience than I had first thought. It was because of the acute feelings of emotion I was still experiencing, which was the residue that remained within my body. I am not normally an emotional person, so these strong emotions were like a calling. I asked my Nun Guide for some explanation.

Her words to me were:-

There are many humans who reach a point within their emotional nature and also their mental nature, where all avenues of reason have been explored. A person comes to a point of despair as they are overcome with emotional impotence, where nothing seems to help or can be done, or there are no ready answers.

This is when the mind has become muddled and cannot see clearly. It is at these times that the human should contact the spirit within, which in turn connects to the godhead. Here is where the illumination is for the asking, and where the consciousness of human souls may fill up with light, to re-vitalise and light up all those who are muddled in mind and emotion.

These are times of great change, both for the individual and for the group and for the planet. In dealing with changing circumstances of the physical, we remind you that the physical is the reflection of that which is taking place within you. It is a fact of earthly life that you create the turmoil without, because of the turmoil within.

So if you are a person who has encountered turmoil recently in your daily life and living, look inwards to see if the circumstances are mirrored within. Try to calm yourself first, so you may see clearly. From then on, you can walk straight and true, knowing that you can draw strength from your spirit guides and brethren whom you are aware of, and also from those you have yet to meet.

The path of earthly life is not an easy road to travel. Much of the time it is like a cobbled path and very hard on the feet. As you know, the meridian lines of the body form, end in the feet, so if your earthly road is indeed stony, it will reflect upon the feet which are a mirror image of all your internal organs. This you can understand and also the fact that physical diseasments can occur, because of the external events having an effect upon the internal constitution of the individual.

You have been given these recent experiences so you will remember what it feels like, when someone asks for your assistance. You will know that in addition to the practical advice and positive thoughts to show others the way, it will also be necessary for the spirit to be engaged.

This is of paramount importance, for without the strength of spirit, the inner knowing and conviction of 'all will be well' will be lost, as the affect upon the person who is experiencing despair, may be to abandon their hold on life itself. The surety of spiritual strength to provide the inner will and purpose towards recovery should never be underestimated.

*Those who **hold the light**, those who hold the faith, can be seen to be a part of the world but not of the world.*

This enables a human to navigate the earthly fields of life and living, without taking upon him or herself undue debris.

By standing within the healing light, all is purified, all is cleared and cleaned.

- o *A New Start.*

- o *A New Day.*

- o *A New Being.*

Live and love the life with all its variations.

It is a wonderland of experience.

Unite with Christ,

Love God.

Blessings upon you.

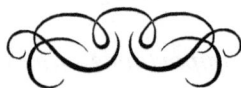

Chapter 21

Arthur Findlay College, Stansted, Essex. UK

Course: Advanced Mediumship Intensive Training Week.

Course Tutor: - Janet Parker

Tutors:
Simon James
Reverend Brian Robertson
Paul Jacobs
Simone Key
Thelma Francis
Brenda Lawrence

After I had received a contact with my Nun Guide at the healing session on 15th July 2008, I was impressed to contact the Arthur Findlay College about the course starting the following week. I found out there was one place left, so I booked myself on this course to provide me with mental physiotherapy, while I waited for the medics to arrange a course for my physical physiotherapy.

I had wanted to go to a healing retreat that was local and did not involve a great mileage. I knew by attending this week I would receive healing by virtue of the wonderful energies that are created at this site. It seemed I was meant to attend this course, as a number of coincidences had provided directions to this event. I booked in at reception and deposited my cases upon the bed nearest to the window in the room allotted. When I had been told I would be in a three bed room I instinctively knew which room it was to be, as another of my friends had occupied this room, last April when I had attended the college.

I went down stairs to retrieve something I had left in the car and another lady was just booking in at reception. We got into conversation and I found out she was to be my room mate. It also transpired that she was the lady who would be working with me in a few weeks time at our local church open day. I had never met this lady before but knew her name. She also knew mine. We both knew Ralph our Church President who was the organiser of the church open day.

As the students arrived they were asked to see the course organiser Janet Parker who would take our names and details to allocate us into the various groups. I was placed with Simon James who had arrived from Canada with Minister Brain Robertson.

During the week I learnt that Simon James and Paul Jacobs had been the two last students of Gordon Higginson, the father of spiritualism, who had passed to the higher life in 1987 and who had worked throughout his life promoting spirit on earth. During the week I received words from Gordon Higginson as I had the last time I had visited this college. At 4.30 pm that afternoon we were all assembled, tutors were introduced and an outline of the work sessions was given to us.

I met my third room mate, a lovely lady of eighty years young. I hope to be as fit and able as she, when I am her age, as she put us all to shame. We had much in common, as we both wrote and received channelled writings from spirit. After each days classes were ended, we were both engaged with homework, channelling from spirit, while our other roommate was occupied with spirits in the bar. This week was one of the best I have experienced as the standards were at their highest. The organisation was superb and the calibre of the lectures was first class. I received the best training to date and enjoyed the wonderful company of the overseas students, who had come from as far as Australia, USA, Canada, Belgium, Holland, Denmark & Switzerland. I made new friends and said hello to those I already knew. The energies of the week were at full throttle as seen from the channelled scripts produced in between classes and lectures.

Day One
26/07/08

Spirit dialogue:-

Here we are again, under the roof of the Arthur Findlay College. Your last visit here was a choppy ride as the vibrations were bouncing up and down with the mix of humans that attended that weeks' course. Today at midsummer, the mix of humans is again diverse due to the multicultural content and includes those who have travelled long distances to the college to experience the high octane energy of the teaching and training activities taking place, to give you the experience of greater connections to spirit.

It is at a place like the Arthur Findlay College that spirit can draw close with ease and action a response from tutors and visitors alike. Many times the guides and spirit teachers have waited for such groups to assemble, so that certain instruction and information can be transmitted to their human subjects. When a place of excellence heralds the forth coming of prime information and knowledge, it goes without saying that humans will take a greater notice, than if that same information had been transmitted from their neighbour or friend. By coming from an objective source, information can carry greater significance than otherwise would be the case.

The colour of orange/peach is brought around you, to give the vitality and warmth for the week ahead. Enjoy and learn in a more relaxed and leisurely manner, as you now have no worries to distract or deflect the concentration and connection. Know that your guides are assembled and will use this occasion to relay the nature of the work ahead. You already have sensed that the international scene beckons you, by the flavour of your fellow students attending this course. It is only when you realise that other countries do not have such facilities for training and development that the Arthur Findlay college supplies, that you realise how fortunate you are, to have such a place not very far from your own Centre of Light.

Do not strain or try any exercise that feels at odds with your psyche. Discriminate in all things. Remember that which suits one person may not necessarily suit another, and your vehicle needs to remain a free zone. The world of messages is always fraught by the calibre of energies abounding. You reach the angelic realms easier than maintaining a link with the human fraternity. This is because your future work will necessitate direct messages from higher realms, to relay truth and knowledge to the masses and not just personal messages to the few.

The earth world becomes smaller as the greater the communications network is displayed and opened fully. Be vigilant about others using your energies as there are always those who would enlarge their egos for self purposes. Make contacts and genuine friends far and wide from all those who will support you and your work. Work methodically, diligently and you will have no regrets upon your stay. Most of all enjoy the uplifting healing energies and the greater gear of faster vibrations as you enter into the colourful energies amassing for your total immersing and delight.

God Bless you.....Your Crusader, Guardian and Guide.

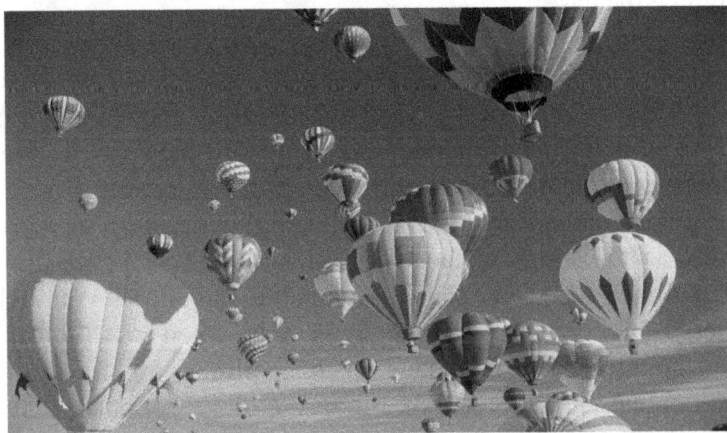

Uplifting Energy

Day Two
27/07/08

Tutor: Simon James

Spirit dialogue:-
We in spirit are gathered here to manipulate the energies between the smaller and larger groups operating this week. The tutors are geared to provide a structure for your work pattern and training, but it is we, of spirit who are lining up the knowledge, messages and information, to be imparted throughout this week.

It is surprising that in each group the dynamics are complex. Yet it is a lesson in brotherhood that so many from different countries or origins, can assemble together with like minds and attitudes to life and living of the spirit.

All are seekers, young and old. All are teachers as each relates to another and something new is learnt. Allow the blending of spirit to take place, so your own inner spirit can shine through. This way your whole being will shine from within and any care or worry can be suspended for the time you are here.

Look for the flow as your Crusader and Nun draw close. Your Crusader is your link to the White Brotherhood and the forward movement in humanities future, and your Nun is your personal link to the Angelic realms where the healing rays are present and can soothe and purify the soul form, from any debris accumulating in the denser spheres.

To travel up and down the spectrum of existences requires a strong constitution. If you happen to inhabit the midway section, you will find that the journey lower, into denser realms requires protective clothing, as you would expect to wear if the climate was cold, wet or snowy. Once appropriately clothed, you would feel comfortable, as you would have been kitted out for the environment into which you have travelled.

It is not unlike your world that has many places of different climates, which require certain changes to the form body in order to acclimatize the being into that particular place.

Similarly, if you journey to the higher realms, the light becomes much brighter and just like it is when you journey to a hot country, you shed some of the clothing and outer trappings to be freer and move au natural. Like any country hot or cold, you adapt to the new circumstances that prevail.

As with various cultures of different countries, the ways of humans differ in their relationships to others. You will find in the spirit realms similar sections of differences, as all variations of ideologies are reflected in the etheric being, so that souls returning home can find their own familiar place with ease.

The Cosmic Lords can wield the power rays to accommodate most eventualities, so a soul who is lost and needs to re-connect to its cosmic awareness, may find itself in a colour frame and undergoing a training course of enlightenment, to assist the inner recognition to truth and realisation.

The levels and understanding of spirit are mirrored in your earth world, if you have eyes to see. The simpleton understands as does the intellectual. All those in between are those who grasp just a little bit of the whole, and are continually asking questions of how and why?

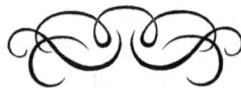

Day Two
Mother Mary

Spirit dialogue:-
Mother Mary stands with outstretched hands, to gather in love, all human kind that assembles to experience the mother glow of love, which emanates from such a high source of purity.

Mother Mary is chief administrator to the angelic host, who are engaged in all directives of help and healing. Today Mother Mary is concerned with the balancing of emotions and health of those students who would become channels and spoke persons for the spirit realms. Our Mother is gentle and all knowing, as she understands the psyche of females and those who think as females do. Many who are born of the male gender are thrown into a female role, to test the mechanics of form in physical living, as part of their long life experiences.

Many who have incarnated as soldiers or priests come to elect to reincarnate as a male again, but they need the more gentle vibrations of a female. A way to gain these feminine attributes is by adopting the nurturing process for children, or those adults that remain children because of mental retardation or growth inhibition. There are many males who are more female orientated inside of themselves, and may show this aspect of their nature in the avenues of creative arts, music, singing and teaching. Often these sensitive males are misunderstood, as they display gentleness in all things and show love at every opportunity, often befriending the orphan or refugee.

In modern times, there are many women who want to be men and they can be seen taking on the role and activities usually associated with males. Many of these women have lived past lives of suppression and need to exert their male side of personality in order to equate the persona overall.

Some of these women are abandon wives and through circumstances, have to take on the responsibilities that traditional male roles would have undertaken. In these cases, the strength of character is being evoked and the learning of self abilities is brought to the surface. Being mother and father is a role often required, so again the male and female natures are required in equal measure.

Mother Mary understands the female nature and influences all those who have a need to express gentle strength and fortitude. Through love, can the understanding come. In love and surety will the rearing of children be given to bring forth a resilient generation of self sufficient adults, who can operate and demonstrate both sides of their nature in perfected unity. It is only when individuals go through some particular disturbance or problem area, that the sight and senses can clearly see the lessons learnt and the value of the recent experiences, to the overall journey of the material life.

Both the genders are in need of the help and healing that Mother Mary offers. At times of great stress, a male and female will remember their childhood and automatically turn to their mother or her equivalent. Through the mothers of present incarnations the Mother Mary shows her influence, for it is in the nurturing of humans that they are brought through troubled times, so they may actuate their potential and realise the purpose of their life blueprint.

Always the human is searching, not always consciously knowing that which he seeks. As soon as Mother Marys love is given, the human glows in response. It is the connection to the spirit realms that the human seeks. He has searched without to find that the connection comes from within, as each soul **holds the light** of spirit and through spirit via spirit above, can the connection be made to God the Creator in whose creation we live, breath and exist.

Mother Mary is always urging humans to look after the children. Many women today are prepared to look after additional children as their maternal instincts are strong and extend to those in less fortunate circumstances. Many children are in desperate circumstances due to the displacement of peoples. In addition there are indiscriminate couplings when irresponsibility is present in both male and female.

Mankind as a species must take on the responsibility of his brother and sister, whose circumstances are not as good as their own. Wherever possible, loving hearts must heal the bridge of separation and humans everywhere must reel in the ties, to the misplaced, misappropriated, mistreated and misfiled.

The future generation is the target to heal, as it is your futures you are ensuring by the actions and attentions of today. If you aspire to perfection, you must engage in the practical issues of life and living, to bring about the betterment of the human condition.

By contributing in someway, by focusing on some particular aspect that applies to you, then know you are engaged in good work. For all work concerning the administration of others is part of Gods great ministry.

If humans understand this, then they can appreciate the work of the Angels who take directive from Mother Mary in matters of nurturing and growth of the young, and also the healing of rifts in relationships, to bring families together in loving unity.

God bless you.

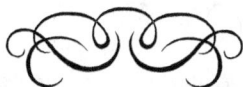

Day Three
Gordon Higginson.
28/07/08

Hello again my earth scribe – back at the Arthur Findlay College.

You notice how many use my method of connecting to spirit and then ask to whom the communication is focused?

This method enables the student to make the spirit connection and in doing so, strengthens personal links to spirit so that you can register within your own being the different energies relayed, as they play upon the scale of registered notes of your personal vehicle of expression which is you.

Like a piano, the student musician has to learn how to co-ordinate the notes and octaves, both in the left hand and right hand, so the whole spectrum of notes can be covered if the tune played requires a large or small expanse of energy wave. You are the conductor so you can manage the orchestra of vibrational notes played, and determine what interpretation is appropriate. Much can be learnt by this method, tune, tempo, volume and stimuli.

A spirit personality will resonate with the notes and form the tune played, so you will know the contact. Practice is the key to improved performance and it is at the Arthur Findlay College that the creases of ones mediumistic suit can be pressed and shaped into the garb necessary for public demonstrations. It is wise to dress appropriately for the occasion as this sets up the intent to validate your appointment with spirit. You are privileged to be associating with my own students who remember the trials and tribulations they encountered when I was chief tutor.

I was strict but fair and always I strived to give my students the understanding necessary to recognise their own spirit within. Humans make things difficult when in fact they are easy.

When the human vehicle is vibrating at the correct note frequency, then the spirit world can flood the channel with knowledge and information of the same frequency vibration.

*Students may receive bits and pieces as their connection goes up and down or in and out of the spiritual sphere. The experienced or mature medium will be able to **hold the light** and power, so spirit can flow the information and knowledge with ease and accuracy. Therefore your aim is to perfect the vehicle of expression that is you, to grow your antenna. Tune into the spirit station and the broadcasts will commence. Learn, Listen and Enjoy*

Thank you scribe.

Day Four
Angel Wings
29/07/08

Angel wings are shown to denote the presence of the Angels who come to assist humans in their earthly living life. Whatever we do as humans upon the earth, Angels are standing by to help and assist when asked or called. Angels can multitask and can be present in many locations at any one time.

When humans assemble in groups for development activities, the Angels rejoice as they see the human heart glow with additional light at the anticipation of connecting to the world of love and light. It is here where both humans and angels can converse. It is here where the souls of humankind can fly free. It is here where the healing light shines bright for many are in need of balance and harmony within their vehicles or body form of expression. Your body form as it is seen in energy terms is always in a state of flux and change, as the life energies move, dance, still and change tempo, at every given circumstance of the physical, emotion or mental experience.

From the high vibrations of personal achievements to the lows of disappointments, the energy spectrum plays its tunes. You can say that as the Angels create the music of the heavenly spheres, humans also create by their very being, the tunes of physical life.

Human musical vibrations are like a big brass band that can blast the sounds far and wide, but can also be gentle and caressing in their softness and approach. Each set of tuneful vibrations or sounds can affect the energy centres of body forms. If a human is suffering from lethargy due to illness or accident, the raising sounds of certain musical renditions will have a most encouraging and uplifting effect. This is an example given to show the benefit of how the sound notes can be used to alter consciousness.

As you think so you are. Energy follows thought. You are all creators of yourselves and can develop self mastery over your physical form, by the use of all the energy centres relating to the seven vehicles of human form expression. As you sit for meditation you listen to the recordings of Angel music of choirs, to take you into the peace and tranquillity of the quiet mind. Here you can rest the body and mind and bring the balance and harmony into your being, to equalise the physical body mechanism for the start of each day.

The journey to the world of love and light.

Your Angel Guide draws near and you see his light shinning from the other side of the road. You stand one side and your Angel Guide on the other side, facing one another. You are both standing on the edge of the super highway leading to the world of love and light. Yet at this moment, all you are aware of is the light emanating from your Angel Guide. You feel a yearning, a drawing towards your Angel Guide who beckons you to him. You do not know how. You are in the physical body and he is of the spirit.

He smiles and says to you,

Let go of your consciousness and allow your focus to join with me, so we may travel on this road to heaven. You will be safe as I will guide you. Your physical body will be safe as you can leave it by the side of the road to rest, until your consciousness and inner being returns to it. So come with me and we will journey to the land of love and light, so I may show you the delight and glory of your heavenly homeland.

As my Angel Guide was talking I realised my inner self had parted from my physical body and had manifested upon the road, this super highway that was leading to the light world ahead. As I drew near the centre of the road, my Angel Guide joined me, to hold my hand firmly as we turned to face ahead, toward the light. I became aware of others like me, holding hands with their guides, to form a procession along this highway. The light of each Angel Guide shines brightly to illuminate the roadway. The light forms a continuous line of light which connects to an enormous ball of a brilliant light globe, which seems to centre itself at a crossroads or intersection, where many roads converged to a central point.

I saw the lines of light converge and disappear within this light globe. As I approached the outer limits, the floodlight defused all around, to engulf the many thousands of heavenly host all converging towards this central place. Each Angel was accompanying a human soul consciousness, who were all willing to sample the light world. We were ushered to a grand auditorium on the lines of a large golden stadium or amphitheatre. Here we were assembled for a Great Lord of Light to transport us up into the next dimension.

I became aware of a labyrinth of light tunnels, like a space station construction of transparent tubes, connecting the dimensions of existence. Elevators were transporting personnel back and forth to intersections and it was at one of these intersections that we were assembled.

In our case we were all visitors, so we were accompanied one to one, by an Angel Guide who normally was able to travel at will. Because of the nature of this occasion, it being such a large group of visitors, a special time or appointment had been arranged, just like you would do, when booking an aeroplane ticket or train ride.

Suddenly I became aware of an even brighter light coming amongst us. Glowing golden white, this Angelic being came to direct us. As we stood there, the whole place was transported upwards. Sounds were heard as we ascended into the land where Angels dwell. All was golden. All was glowing. I found myself transported to a mystical garden with a fountain at its centre. This was a golden fountain with water flowing into the pool surrounding it, where water lilies formed a circle. I knew this was the fountain of eternal renewal, and knew this fountain and place held magical powers. I must have questioned this, as immediately I saw older people, crippled souls with their Angel carers who had brought them to this place for healing.

I knew that many of these people were newly departed souls for all were wrinkled with age and infirmity. As each came to this fountain, they were given water to drink from the healing pool. I watched as each one underwent a transformation, to become once again young and wholesome. The beauty of their spirit was displayed to show them at their best, as they were, when at the height of their physical appearance and health. I was witnessing the renewal of forms as they drank in the divinity of the light essence that forms the golden glow of a cosmic being, which shows its spiritual expression. As soon as this transformation had taken place, there were thanks given to the Angel Guides who then led the souls to the elevators I had become aware of, situated to one side of this garden of renewal. I knew that this was a clearing station that was being shown to the visitors of earth, so we would know the procedure when first returning to the spiritual sphere. The earthly trappings had been left behind, but the soul body was still expressing itself in its former appearance.

Once the treatment had worked by filling the soul with soul light, the ashes of form expression disintegrated, to fall away. The soul light form is then shown in its natural beauty and healthy state.

This cleaning and purifying process is required to eliminate any contamination from one sphere to another, prior to the journey of the soul to its rightful place, according to its vibrational note and sound. This is why I could hear the sounds from the multitude of souls as Angelic tunes of rejoicing were heralding the joyous reunion between loved ones, for celebrations are regular events when spirits reunite. I was taken to a country scene where a mother and father were waiting for their son. I saw a young man draw close, who recognised this couple and all hugged and cried at this reunion.

After a while I saw the three of them looking radiant. They then turned towards earth with sadness and regrets, as I saw a scene on earth where another couple were mourning the recent loss of a beloved son. I knew that the son who had died on earth due to a fatal illness, was the son just returned to spirit. He was in fact the true son of the couple in spirit, but had been born as a grandson within the same family unit. A physical life for a short period of time was sought, to fulfil karmic obligations. The scene on earth was of distraught parents from the recent loss of their son, but you could see that this event was a lesson for them and their other children, as their future would somehow be enhanced because of this experience.

Another scene beckoned me. It was a joyous celebration by Angels and Cherubs playing musical instruments. Many were sitting around listening to this concert. The Cherubs were experimenting with the notes to bring forth new sounds and melodies from the inspirational sources. I could see an avenue connecting to the earth and to a group of university students. The Angel music was being relayed as inspiration to this group of earth students, who were trying to recreate in composition, the interpretation of the music of the spheres. When a new melody was mastered, there was great rejoicing both in the spirit world and earth world.

Another scene caught my attention as my guide showed me the way to what looked like a large church gathering. This was a more formal setting where Angels and aspiring human souls gather to pay homage to their Lord Creator. I knew that these meetings of formal church gatherings were ceremonies to bring greater understanding to those existing on the many dimensional levels, which need understanding of how the heavenly energies and vibrations work.

At first there was communion with the great light, which brought extra power and strength to the proceedings. Then the light power or Christ light was beamed forth, and I could see the lines of power light shinning forth in many directions to the earth world, to touch and influence those who were also attending the churches, chapels, centres and gatherings for the purposes of greater enlightenment.

It was interesting to realise that the Spirit Church seemed constructed on Christian lines, which was acceptable to my way of thinking, but the connections to earth could be seen to encompass a diversity of Groups, Assemblies, Churches, Mosques and meeting places with communal intent. I became aware of a group of native Indians from South America living primitively. The closeness to their natural surroundings had brought them the understanding of the universal spirit, which for them could be seen in the animals and vegetation of their habitat.

In addition they were in touch with the Earth Angels to such a degree, that they were nearer to the etheric builders and divas of nature, than other humans of more advanced cultures. I was then shown the average man and women whose brief understanding of spiritual matters is gained in childhood and which comes to the forefront at times of stress and strain in the earthly life.

These are the gatherings to celebrate births, deaths and marriages where the impact of another dimension suddenly presents itself for consideration. A wake up call is brought to the average human within the lesser world. Again I was made aware of the counter part in eastern countries where life in the village or countryside is harsh.

The assemblies amongst the simple folk were less formal but again the consideration was geared to those times when necessity prevailed. Unlike their western brothers, the eastern cultures are very strong and many of the spiritual ceremonies have been incorporated into daily life rituals. This forms a connection on a daily basis, so the disposition of such humans realise a greater understanding of the spirit within, even though they may not have the opportunities to express it to others, outside of their immediate families.

To many of the regular church goers who are seen to be stuck in a rut, like a record whose needle is stuck in a grove, and therefore the record keeps revolving going nowhere, this message was given. *Break out of your present and comfortable lifestyles and find the light within.*

Again I was directed to the many sensitive humans abiding in every land, who are operating alone, outside of formal organisations. These are the individuals with soul light that is shinning outwards for all to see. Little by little the lights are gravitating to each other and amalgamating together with some souls travelling great distances, to be able to commune with like kind. When enough are joined together, they send out a tremendous light, which is seen like a beam entering the cosmic universe. So direct is this light, it reaches up to the highest zenith of being. This light is gaining strength and surety as the many light beings presently incarnate are uniting in understanding and are using the earth networks of love and light to matrix together, (Internet) so that their collective broadcasts of light, penetrates all barriers and enables a straight line of connection to the Godhead, to the Master Creator.

This evocation of thoughts direct to the Godhead has brought the Celestial Host nearer to the planet earth, as more and more are challenging the established religions and are connecting directly to source. The requests are always for help and healing as the negativity of religious fervour increases to challenge the spearhead of ascension. This is why the Angels, Ascended Masters and enlightened humans forming the White Brotherhood are working to bring about the greater awareness of the spirit in each human soul.

We all have responsibility to our bothers, so each of us must use what ever means available to us, to bring light and love into the hearts of all misguided souls. Follow not your mortal brother but listen to the spirit within. Follow the light beams for direction to take you onto the spiritual highway, for it is this road that leads to the heavens and to the world of love and light. Natural laws will sort the wheat from the chaff. Where there is unrest, send loving thoughts if you are not directly involved. Concentrate upon your own life and refine your own qualities first before trying to influence others.

Know that the spiritual hierarchy are ever close by and know also that love is the determining factor to all things. Be happy and love the earthly life to the full. Take on board the wisdom gems, given in word or print. Accept what resonates within you as true, and try to put good relations into practice. Form your brotherhoods and sisterhoods by the groups or organisations you assemble and remember to work in truth always, so light and love will walk with you as your Angel Guide makes sure you keep travelling upon the super highway.

This is so you may enter the labyrinth of light in your final days and realise all you have learnt and seen in those journeys of visitations, when given a glimpse of the Angel Host in the heavenly spheres.

Remember the times when you journeyed into the spirit realms. Remember that the light from the world of the Christ consciousness is always available to those who can reach up to touch the stars. Remember the Angel Guide by your side, who will hold your hand when needed.

Spread your knowledge wide and true. Impart your experiences for others to know. Love the living life you have chosen, and by joining the two worlds together, may you express and demonstrate that greater love and light, which comes from the spirit world, your true home and heritage.

God Bless you......Your Angel Guide.

Day Five & Six

Alana
30/07/08 & 31/07/08

I am Alana your light being from the world of the celestial cosmos. I come to spend time with you as your light beacon has indicated contact at this time. You are sending your beam of light to attract communications so here I am to converse with you.

As before I am still teaching the young souls from both the Angelic and Human worlds who attend my class for light absorption, to grow in knowledge by attunement to the world of love and light where the illumined minds and souls reside. I have also been visiting the sleeping souls to try and awaken them to the divine light of living. There are many humans who do not believe in life continuance and think when their life on earth is ended, that they will rest and not have to be anymore.

Many souls have issues unresolved and we in spirit often induce the sleep state so a soul can take time within their minds to resolve the impediments of their thinking. It is to these I administer, for when in the sleep state renewal and healing can take place.

The soul can be taken on inner journeys so it can be made ready for its grand awakening within the spirit world. Often a soul returns to spirit in a confused state and a little sleep to resolve issues outstanding and to bring the mind into the quiet is all that is required. The pull of the great light from our Master Creator is present and plays on soul energy fields to bring that soul to its proper resonance within the great universal life.

It is like being given a stimulus to wake you up, when you are comfortable in your dream state and do not want to wake up from your safe haven. It is not that you are afraid, but more because we in spirit have induced a euphoric state, which is very appealing to the soul, particularly when mesmerised by the wonderful light displays we use to align the energies. An awakening soul is a very beautiful event. The reality of a new homeland where your dear ones reside is a powerful drawing force.

The many activities within the heavenly spheres are truly endless, for existence is never ending and evolvement of souls continuous. Life is eternal. Spirit does not have a clock, so time does not apply in the same sense as you know it. In spirit, events occur by actual progression of endeavour. Where time does apply is when the groups are transmitting specific power and energy to the earth world, and this involves the alignment of specific power lines of energy, where the timing in earth terms is relevant.

You know or have heard about the coming changes to your planet and predictions from Earths predecessors, have indicated a timescale when this will come to pass. The time for spirit is governed by celestial moments and the cycle alterations of energy times as a result of movements through the evolutionary circle. There is more to your zodiac than you suppose, for the colour wheel is like our clock. Each segment is an age in your terms and in each age the journey of the creations must find its way from the outer edges of the circle of influence, to the central point where the creative source resides. This is mirrored in your own microcosmic creative process of the human species.

The elders of our universe have travelled the wheel of life in its turning many times, so that is why the ancients are all knowing. We who are light beings of angelic form, know about such matters but have not experienced all things yet, as we are engaged directly with the lives and evolution of mankind.

It is what our Lord Almighty wishes, and it is our service to him so that this work continues unabated. If you think that when you vacate the physical form, you and your existence ends, then think again. The heavens never rest in the great creative process. We in spirit welcome the many humans who are willing to help us in our work. Many humans have been light beings in former existences and have elected to assist human kind by taking on the physical form and incarnating within an earth family. Often the ability to touch the souls of humankind is made easier when concurrently of the physical world. If you look to your history books you will find some wonderful examples of human life where the life itself has left a legacy of meaning and purpose.

The life lived has helped change the thinking or living conditions of human life in some way. The service has been given. The purpose fulfilled. In your present world there are many angelic souls walking the globe as humankind. These are special people whose purpose is to enlighten and uplift those around them, and even enter the governing bodies of your organisations, to bring about change in its wider sense or meaning.

We who are light workers bring enlightenment to all we touch. It is our work to educate, bring knowledge and understanding to those we reach. Encourage where we can to those who are on the path, but may need a helping hand from time to time. We send love to you as we need a communicative channel, so more humans may become aware of our influence.

Many call for help and assistance but do not recognise the presence of their helpers or the subtle help that is often given but is often missed or overlooked, because of a lack of awareness or perception. We send love so you may sooth the edges of frayed nervous energy, as students when learning can become frustrated when their endeavours fall short of expectations.

Everyone needs help at some time, so do not be afraid to ask. By asking, you show your own recognition of the fact that you are now ready to proceed to engage your new activity. I have to go now as my fellow workers are assembling in a gathering to energise anew, for we too have to find accord to the renewable energies for the continuance of our work.

We are thankful that there are those on your earth planet who know about energy, about building the powerhouses from your earth dimension to provide the colour streams that circulate your globe. If you did but know, there is an army of light workers all busy and working to generate the light vibrations out of the inert substance and life forms unawakened. It is part of this age of ascension where we have begun a new segment of the colour wheel to bring the attributes of Aquarius into the lives of the many existences, within this colour spectrum of the now. In your meditations and prayer sessions the beams of light and love are released into the universal void. This energy amalgamates at the depots which stores and holds such energy, for positive energy uses.

The energy generated is not stored long as the whole purpose of generating love and light on beams of energy, is to use this power where it is needed most. Like all power stations upon your world, a regulated flow of energy is required to provide the necessary applications for living and welfare. Similarly, we in spirit need to replicate the energy supplies and make sure it is sent or provided where the need is great. Often prayers and thoughts are sent out for a specific purpose or with intent to a specific person, place or occurrence.

These directives are forwarded to their destination forthwith, like your express postal service, but as you know your light networks make communications much faster, so we employ our own light network to super track all the messages, thoughts and healing energy from source to recipient.

This is the communications web network that provides transference within your awareness. You know this as your radio waves of audibility are used, transmitted and received in long and short wave lengths. Our network exists within the colour spectrum of faster vibrations, for always we use colour energy where we can, as it provides avenues within the light spectrum in which we operate.

God Bless You Always ...Alana.

Day Seven
01/08/08
Gordon Higginson
Hello again,

'You have enjoyed this week I know and seen many of the students work using my methods and witnessed the results. I am pleased to leave my mark upon so many in the furtherance of service to our spirit friends. Now that I am one of them I teach from this side on how best to contact and provide information that can be clearly understood. No more days in the cupboard, I was a young student who had exacting teachers as my own mother was a hard task master and when young I had to deal with the conflict of personal emotions as well as the emotions felt by those in spirit that needed to contact their loved ones on earth.

I bless my mother for her strong faith in my abilities as on many occasions I would have jacked it all in. As you may know my life was engaged with spirit and spiritualism, as my job became more important in holding together the many mediums that provided the necessary communications between the two worlds. Equating the needs of spirit and man often conflict, as any medium will know. The spirit comes first, for it is where you all started from and is pure in its essence of divinity. Man wishes to covet and contain in his fear of loosing control.

Trust spirit, love spirit. Allow spirit to influence and you will see there are no boundaries where spirit or human souls abound. We are all one and should love one another. This needs to be demonstrated by putting into action fair and steady policies to apply to the physical workings of mediumship in all its guises. More and more students are seeking direction and training.

The channels are lined up and it is like an airfield. You need to fill up with fuel to propel the aircraft into the air. Many have the knowledge to fly, but do not know how to fuel up their vehicle for take off. The techniques of mediumship enable the filling up of the vehicle and once airborne the limits of flying free are endless'.

God Bless you Scribe.

Day Seven
Contacting the Source.
01/08/08

The meditation to contact the source within began with concentrating on the breathing, to take us to the centre of our being. The class tutor had a melodic voice and soon I could no longer register her words, I could only make out the hum of her voice.

I became aware of a Red Indian standing in the centre of our circle. He was wearing a full headdress of white feathers and was dressed in a light buckskin suit with a jacket that had long sleeves and was decorated in leather and bead adornments.

On his right arm was perched a large white bird. This bird was the size of an eagle with eyes of a hawk and yet its colour was representative of a white dove of purity and peace and its soft feathers were reminiscent of a wise old snowy owl. The bird was as wise as an owl, but needed the eyes of a hawk and the strength of an eagle, to forward the energy power building within this circle. His mission was to carry the powerful energies of healing love, light and peace to the four corners of the world.

As I looked around I saw all twelve of us within the physical meditation circle as Red Indian braves with our heads bowed in reverence to this high Shamanic Lord and teacher appearing as the Red Indian Chief of all nations. I became aware of him swinging a large diamond crystal, to and fro. The action reminded me of a catholic priest swing the orb of incense at a service. Likewise the diamond crystal was cascading vapour streams of stardust to each of us, the braves of the circle.

There was a perfume mist building up from this enormous crystal diamond pendant as it moved back and forth. As the movement continued, the vapours and mist of sparkling stardust scattered with the movements, and began swirling around each and every one of the twelve persons within the circle. As it did so, it was filling us all up with light essence of star fragrance. As I looked again at the Shamanic Lord, he became the Christ administering to his twelve disciples.

I knew that this central entity was the anointed one, who has taken many guises over the ages, to head all the nations, the great tribes and world religions. As this realisation occurred to me, I saw his face change to that of the Buddha, Krishna, and Abraham, endorsing the heritage of the central source which stretches back to the beginning of time and creation itself. The great wheel of the colour zodiac was presented with the central core of power flowing outward to form the colour reel of existence and creation.

To the central core where the source is found. Each segment of the colour reel is the arc of passage that each soul must take in its life existence. Connecting to the core of your being, is the connection to the very source of power, light and love where is found our Great Creator, that **G**reat **O**mnipotent **D**eity we call **GOD**.

--------------------o------------------

At the closing ceremony within the sanctuary at the Arthur Findlay College, the candles were lit and prayers and thoughts offered to the Godhead. The music raised vibrations upwards so evoking the meditative state. I saw another group, a circle of nuns, with my own nun guide taking centre stage, as the line of other nuns circled round in time with the musical vibrations.

This was felt by others as a high spiritual presence coming amongst the earth circle of attending students. Pure silver and white patterns of rich filigree artwork of intricate designs were shown. A beautiful vision to close the week of spirit contact when two worlds entwined.

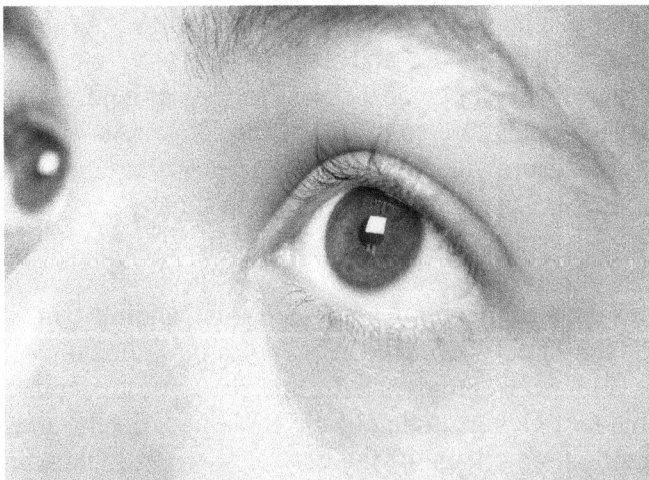

Looking Upwards

Chapter 22.

SAINT AUGUSTINE
08/08/08

In the early hours of the morning, I had awoken and in that half sleep state, I became aware of a priest or monk who sat ready to talk to me. He was of olive skin and dark hair and the name he gave me, was Augustine. He was with me for most of the day until later I found time to sit quietly to hear what he wanted to say.

It is a special day today as it is at this time that the opening to the Christ Consciousness is fully widened to allow the centring of this energy to be a permanently grounded force upon the earth planet as part of the ascension process. The time approaches when the portals of awareness from the celestial high council are opening according to alignments of geometric co-ordinates.

This allows the awareness of the human being to connect with the higher energies without having to bridge the defences that hitherto have impeded direct contact with the central source. The dates of your calendar align with the numerical frequencies. 080808, 090909, 101010, 111111. & 121212.

I draw near you at this time as the energies are again drawing the Christ light into the hearts of humans. I come to help the race in the ascension process to enable the many to recognise the Christ light that is centred within their hearts. It is that loving feeling of knowing that you are at one with the cosmos, the planet and all that abounds and is around you.

The realisation that your spirit is part of that divine nature you call God, the father and creator of all things. From the source of Gods power and love comes all things, comes all understanding, comes all knowing.

You do not have to search for answers when all you need is to find Christs love and light, and merge with his essence to become part of this powerful vibration, and then you will know all things, for all will be clear in sight and understanding. Your faith is strong, when all about you are wavering in doubts. It is for you to relay the words and messages we in the finer world wish to impart. It is important that information is recorded so humans can verify that which is relayed.

In the coming weeks you will see many more humans seeking spiritual answers. More humans will seek solace within the churches, chapels and centres of spirituality. Many will not receive the answers they expect, as the personnel of churches in your country have wandered far from truth. Many will wonder why they are feeling bewildered, or lost or at sea. They feel the quiver of vibrations but may not recognise the source, until a major happening awakens them.

Love your neighbour, for brotherhood and sisterhood is the key to the unity of the species. Look after the less fortunate as all share equal responsibility and cannot isolate themselves from current affairs. The knower's which are your light-workers are drawing near to each other and in joining forces they are signalling the cohesive force which unites all people, where minds and hearts vibrate with notes of harmony.

The main thrust of the army of light-workers has yet to take place, as many more sleepers are to awaken with the influx of energies and especially the Christ white light of love, before the legions can begin to march forth.

Know that as the Christ light begins to be absorbed and reflected upon the planet, the forces of evil flee, as negativity of any kind cannot remain where love and light prevail. You stand on the cusp of a new era where the changes upon your world will be of a daily happening. While there is much disquiet in your living material life, the spiritual aspect of living is beginning to appeal to more humans.

When the false gods of the material life are found to be wanting, the young are quick to seek alternatives, for they are always seeking to learn more as they mature into adulthood. When hearts and minds turn from hate to love, then a transformation will be seen. The light of the world is held in each human heart and needs the key to open it.

Like the flowers in your garden, the summer sun is required to bring nature into maturity. The cosmic sun as the Christ light is now pouring onto your world. Look around you and see the coming bloom of natural growth and beauty where love and light has taken root. The beauty, the wonderment can be seen as the height of attainments are reached, by those who have been able to reach up and touch the zenith of their being.

In times of great change there needs to be a framework for those who would work in service as light-workers. My work on earth left lines of thoughts for prosperity. It was necessary then as the human intellect was not so developed in the masses.

Today I advocate the simple approach, for it is with our hearts that we will feel the movement of energies most, as the Christ light and love takes affect. It is in the healing of others that the energies of Christ should be applied, for many are in need of balance and harmony of the being.

I will carry the Cross of the Lord of Love, to light your way. I will take a benediction in honour of those who aspire to the new era of ascension. Many will find their own connection, through their heart centre, now that the portal of Christ consciousness has opened wide.

It will be easier also for the many to receive guidance direct, and the understanding of spirit and life continuance will become universally accepted. Know that I and many of my brothers in spirit take the Christian services in our attempts to send light energy to the earth groups, where further enlightenment is required. Always we advocate co-operation between groups and fellow humans.

The Angel of the Lord stands straight and true. His great presence brings surety and trust to all those in his service. His light shines for all, to light the way for all humans who are seeking his illumination, so they may be heralded upon the right roadway, where the ascension of human beings is taking place.

The higher selves of human souls are lining up for cohesion with their material counterpart. The duality of being is synthesizing into unity, so that the Christ light can shine though every living heart and soul, so it may shine upon the planet Earth to bring about that transformation into a heavenly habitat, where both Angels and Humans may dwell.

......................Amen

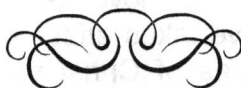

Chapter 23

Concerto of Life
14/08/08

Spirit dialogue:-
The sounds of the orchestra are heard as the rain clouds above herald a summer shower of some magnitude. The notes start by a gentle rendition of sounds as water droplets fall to earth. Outside of a window the droplets slowly slide down the windowpane. The wind blows and a trumpet is heard, followed by some gentle breathing space before the crescendo of a bursting raincloud descends downwards.

The armies of the storm clouds unite in formation as the wind rushes forward in advance of the main thrust of descending water, which pelts down in such fury that the leaves of trees bend with the onslaught. Now the tapping can be heard upon the windows of dwellings as the heavy downpour gets underway.

The water sprites are having a wonderful time as they take this opportunity to reformulate their tactics around natures treasures of natural formations, formed upon the earths surface. It is summertime, but with this dark cloud overhead, it could be winter as it is so dark and grey. The foliage of vegetation is in full display and lavishes this downpour as a refreshing interlude.

This sudden rendition of a heavenly sonata gives way to a more accepted summer symphony that reminds us of the musical masters of old. Their music is still played and used, for the education of the young.

Such was the inspiration relayed at the time of renaissance that there has not been any time since, that could be compared or matched to the quality or quantity of gems, that stirred the musings of mankind. The trumpets and horns sound again, as the downpour lifts from its heavy state, to be gently blown over fields afar. There are trumpets of success and awakening, as after a drenching such as this. All that has been doused is cleaned and refreshed. The earthly spirits of fairies shake their heads of dew and clamber for the dry places under trees and in caves.

Much work takes place once the rain has ceased, as all the vegetation that has taken the onslaught needs tending, so that they may again stand upright in the summer sun. Many of the plants and shrubs will be soaking up the water vapour into their living arms and branches. Much must be stored and treasured, for it is unpredicted when the next round of water showers will occur.

This is the last spurt of nourishment before the harvest ensues. The animals are gathering their hoard for wintertime and gorging upon the fat of the land, to tide them over the lean time ahead. This year will be very lean, as the harvest upon the hedgerows and trees can be seen to be exceptionally lush at this time.

This exhibition of goodness foretells a lean time ahead, so much harvesting must take place now, in preparation. The human populace should also take note, as what applies to the animal and vegetable kingdoms, also applies to the human kind. Mankind often miss the obvious because he has his own agenda and forgets to look at what nature predicts and foretells.

Ignore the signs at your peril, for it is part of the divine system to provide for everyone who has eyes to see, and can read the signs of natures ways, which is Gods way of providing for all his creations.

It is at this time that the portal of the Christ light has opened fully to display the magnitude of light beams shinning upon your earth world. The energy force of light and love is now centred within Mother Earth, who is ready to activate this energy, so all manifestations that form part of her body and surface areas can profit from this awakening to energise anew.

Many humans will find that the time ahead is one of great change as the mixture of energies begin to sort and wrestle for supremacy The consciousness of mankind will have to make a choice. The light workers are those who are gathering together with like mind and purpose, to bring the race of man into the next dimensional awareness.

Through the testing times upon the material level of existence, the souls of human beings are awakening. Many are waking up to the fact that the material life falls short of expectations and fulfilments. This is why alternatives are sought and it is to the spirituality of being, that the spotlight is focused.

It is well known that the eastern philosophies have stood the test of time, as many facets of each line of ideas and knowledge threads have filtered into the minds or psyche of western man. As a result the balance of living in both east and west is in the process of re-balancing. Soon the many will become self aware, and by connecting directly to the source of knowledge, and to the land of love and light, the necessary understanding of self and self being will be more fully understood.

As this becomes widespread, more and more of the populace will seek the qualitative avenues for fulfilment. Many will realise that the life of living continues after the physical body is shed, so many more will want to use the celestial telephones, by engaging a sensitive of mediumistic ability, to relay those loving words direct from relatives now residing in the spiritual realms.

The role of the mediumistic operator will become something like the roles now carried out by the nature spirits who act to liaise between dimensions of existence and reality. To act as a bridge between the dimensions will bring great responsibility, as the standard of attainment and delivery, needs to be of the highest if the same is sought, from the other planes of manifestation.

Know that the elements of nature are ever in a state of flux for creativity and maintenance is an ongoing activity.

We, who draw close to man at this time, are working with our brothers of the White Brotherhood. Likewise this is a time when more will gravitate into groups, when it becomes realised that there is greater influence and power, when amalgamating with others of like mind.

The energies of activity including natures wonders are gathering momentum and cohesiveness. The more evolved that humankind becomes, the more he relies upon the natural processes of nature and his surroundings. In personal awareness the student will find the close association with all things of nature as well of those inherent qualities of colour and attributes found in the vegetable and mineral kingdoms for all is intertwined and interlinked.

The impact of sounds, music, vibrations and rhythms are taking effect to bring the mass of human souls into awakening. It is like seeing an army, which is lying down to form a green carpet, that is suddenly transformed by a heralding of sounds, to realise that they are all sun flowers, and can stand erect with their faces turned upward, to the glowing light of living and the realisation of self being.

Such is the awakening upon the earth planet. There is a need for gardeners of many kinds to nurture these tender souls. Some will be hardy and become the teachers and trainers of tomorrow. Others will need varying amounts of help and assistance to find their personal avenue of expertise to fulfil their mission on the road of living the spiritual life.

Some of the others will show exceptional gifts and talents. These are the souls of great sensitivity which require special handling and care. The young in particular will need guidance for the weight of responsibility may be heavy on the shoulders of such young persons.

It will be to the elders of the race that the students turn for guidance so that they may be steered straight and true, upon the highway of physical and spiritual life that they have chosen, in order to demonstrate the life more abundant, when realising the manifested life, within both the physical and spiritual realms.

We on the spirit side of life are always a thought away. Ever eager to assist when the permission is given for us to help you. We see a little further than you, for we are not clouded in judgement by emotional turmoil when others pull this way and that. We are forever sending thoughts and ideas to those who can make use of our suggestions, for the free will of man is always respected.

To those who are receptive to our influence, we treasure you, for when we find a channel to relay our thoughts and words we can then engage in meaningful dialogue, to help the masses of humans who are floundering in their attempts to live the material life when facing the reconciliation to their inner spirit.

Those who find the material life difficult to handle are those whose soul is awakening. As soon as this process begins there is conflict between the material mind and the intuitive knowing of the inner self. It seems that every step of material life is challenged by some unseen force. This is when you know it is a time of personal choosing. Mans dual nature is at odds with itself when the drive is to unite with the spirit counterpart.

When the choice takes you beyond the conflict so that the hurdle is overcome, then the calm of knowing you now walk the correct pathway is one of upliftment and satisfaction. In all that you do in the living life, the tempo and rhythm of the symphony of liveliness, brings energies to you for you to use and experience.

In realising the material life, in playing your own concerto, you play the many melodies and songs that govern your earthly existence, so that when your time comes to transcend the dimensions, you will know what tune to play, so you may consciously participate in the homeward journey to take you to your spiritual destination.

So all humans should know and appreciated the music of both heaven and earth, for much of life's events are in direct response of some initiated force or energy. You call this cause and effect. This is known as karma which can be positive or negative according to the original intent.

The modern therapy of using positive thinking endorses this maxim. It is also well known and accepted that action follows thought. How many times were you told as a child to think before you act? Many a child has been chastised by its parent for acting without thinking beforehand, as it falls fowl of accepted behaviour or action. It is important that the intent is positive so as to bring about the best attainment possible.

Our advice to all humans is to enjoy companionship. Use your friends to discuss and debate the various issues of human life and living. Where possible, put forward those positive ideas that have practical applications in the now, and work upon other ideas for future implementation. What you cannot do today may well be possible tomorrow for the world as you know it is a changing fast.

The ideas for living a more fulfilling existence are already known within the confines of the human mind. It is putting things into practice that is the challenge of today, for the physical world of earth and the living life upon it, is so diverse that the grounding of energy and ideas into a static form, to bring about manifestation, requires a great deal of energy and effort from human forms.

It is the time and dedication required which translates as sacrifice in personal terms and commitment. Now you can understand why it is, that those who are visionaries are the ones dedicating their whole life to a particular cause or idea. It is from those who are inspired and who take up the banner of righteousness for human progress, that we see the spiritual light shinning forth from their persona.

Many more humans will shine their light for all to see.

The Christ light is the golden light of enlightenment. It is the light of Knowing. It is the light of Unity. It is the Understanding that we are at one with the Great Lord Creator, Our Heavenly Father, that divinity of being we call GOD.

God Bless you ….Amen. The Brotherhood…. Fini - Allegro

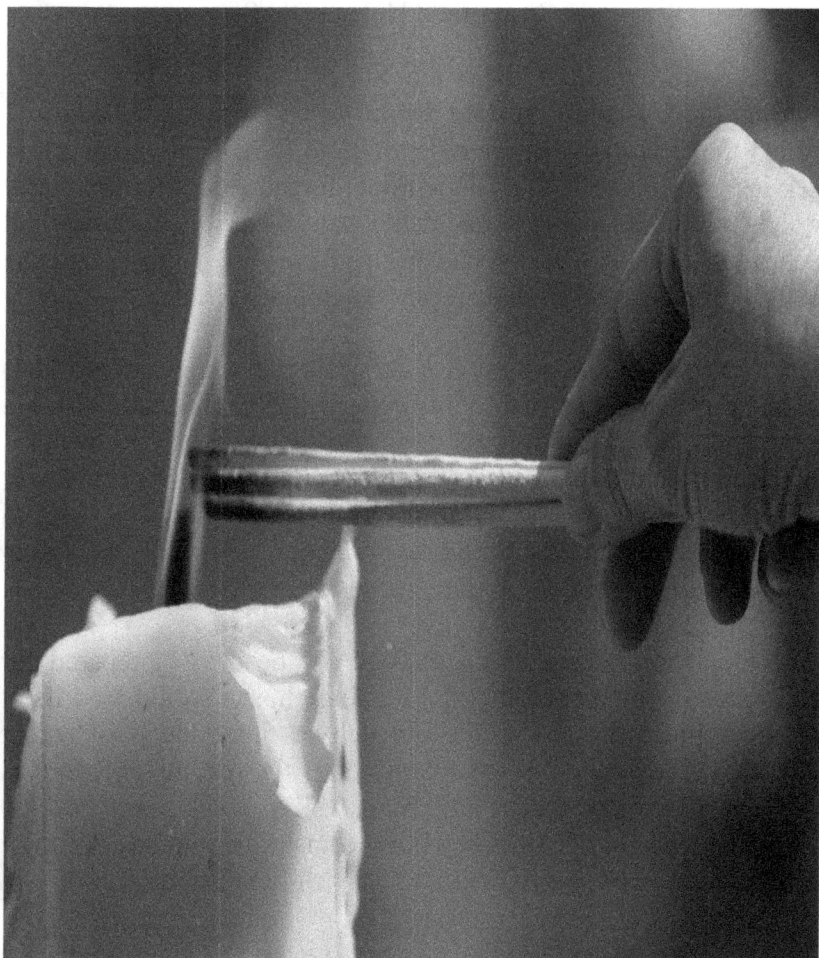

Keep the Light Burning

Chapter 24

Back to Work
Sunday 17th August 2008

Service at Springfield House, Old Stevenage.

I had been invited to take the Sunday Service at Stevenage Springfield House in the Old Town on 17th August 2008, and I found that I was slightly nervous, due to the fact it was the first service I would be taking, since my enforced rest, after my major operation and hospitalization. A few weeks earlier I had attended a healing session where I had been taken on a journey into the spirit realms via the meditative or contemplative state.

I had experienced some aspects of spirit life which I could later recount to others and within this experience there contained some very good insights and truths of spirit life and existence, which I believed would assist and give credence to others. By explaining aspects of spirit life and living it would be possible for others to also realise the same or similar experiences, when they were able to take journeys with their spirit guides and helpers.

This was the theme running through my head as I prepared for this service, so I hoped that the reading chosen would lend itself to the subject chosen, so I could deliver this address of recent experience. I should not have worried, as the reading chosen was the last few pages of Tony Stockwell's book 'The Psychic Detective' where he describes how to make that contact to spirit and take your consciousness into the spirit dimensions.

This lead me to explain, that the best method of spirit contact is via meditation, and that this state of altered consciousness can be attained if a person is receiving healing, particularly if they are of a sensitive disposition.

As this was exactly what I had experienced in recent weeks, it was very appropriate that I could relate a process of attunement from personal experience, and stand there in front of a congregation to relate my experiences in detail.

This was appreciated by the congregation as during the message giving from spirit afterwards, I was able to verify with one lady that she too, had that closeness to her spirit friends, which has enabled her also to undertake journeys into the realms of love and light. This lady also verified her interest in Angels and I was able to confirm that she had two Angels who stood beside her, so she was indeed in good company.

I had been concerned as to the calibre of the messages I would be able to relay as the method of spirit transmitting information to me, has changed over the years. Most students start by receiving clear clairvoyant images which they have to interpret to relay an understandable and comprehensive communication.

Because of my recent health problems and the recent knowledge imparted, that somehow my mediumship would be enhance in some way, I was seeking the clear images that are much easier to work with. What I found was that I was working as of old, receiving very brief impressions but able to relate information which was being accepted straight from my mind and this was new to me, as it was like I had become a loud speaker plugged into a talking source.

This was slightly unnerving as it was more of a case of standing in the power and speaking what ever words were given in my head. I did get one or two No's where the recipient could not place the person described, so I was able to ask for another spirit person who would be recognisable, which became the case, so no one missed out. I did notice that in at least another two messages the contact did not want to be described, but gave other information about themselves so they could be identified.

This was the case for one lady when her father made contact, so I knew he was a person who was more comfortable standing in the background that being upfront. I knew he was her father but he would not show himself to me so I could not describe what he looked like. Instead he made me aware of and injury to his leg which gave him problems thereafter. The lady confirmed this was accurate.

I went to a gentleman who was hard of hearing. His mother wanted to make contact, so we had some fun trying to get him to understand what was being said. Fortunately his daughter was with him. When he was shaking his head and not understanding, she was nodding in agreement. I found this communication hard work and the lady in spirit agreed that her son hadn't change a great deal from when he was young, as he had been hard work then. I voiced this state of affairs and every one burst out laughing finding the whole communication one of upliftment.

I realised that spirit use every opportunity to bring healing in its many forms to those who are in need. Not everyone needs the hands on healing, but everyone benefits from messages given from dear ones in spirit. This service may have seemed ordinary on the surface but it held great teaching and understanding within its deliverance. It seems I am definitely back to work.

Usually at the services at Springfield House, the medium goes home with the lovely flowers used to decorate the altar table for the service. This particular week the lady officer of the church who brings the flowers was kept at home. She had developed a swelling to her face after an insect bite. I missed out on the flowers but took home many appreciated thanks.

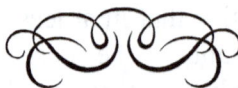

Chapter 25

The Angel of Light.
Healers of All Souls, Letchworth.
21/08/08

Spirit dialogue:-

I stood beside you only yesterday when you were receiving the healing vibrations from your friend and colleague. She told you that she felt me near and described the sensation of feeling so much taller than her usual self.

You saw me with your inner sight, holding the cup of light, so connecting the physical to the etheric realms. You registered the high vibrations of the healing energy which was sent through this connection, and this was verified by your friend who was impressed to move her hands to the appropriate areas for healing.

You should not be surprised when an Angel appears, for when you play music dedicated to Angels you raise the vibrations, and summon those who respond on the equalization of the same notes and call.

We bring the golden light of Christ which is the vibration used for healing the physical form of humans upon the earth world. It is this essence which is within all human hearts and once activated, the healing processes will bring the human form to its optimum healthy state.

Look out for the golden light of your age, for all animated forms which demonstrate this lighted spirit which will be recognizable as souls touched and blessed by that divine spark of God, that goodness which is seen in the purity of being. This is the attained state which angels demonstrate in their revelation to human beings. This is why Angels are seen glowing in countenance. It is because of the divine spark God reveals and manifests within the soul form of the Angel being.

The greater the light force that is seen shinning from within an angelic form, the greater the strength of manifested essence, which registers the nearness to the central source, and which shows itself by colouring all that it touches, in brilliance and glory. Such is the beauty of the celestial bodies of high vibrational notes and purity. This is love in manifested glory and magnificence. It is blinding in its light, it is overwhelming in its emotional content, and it is mind blowing in its splendour of illumination.

To experience the atonement with the highest aspect of your ability and being is to realise the magnificence and magnitude of creation in its being state. **To Be** *- is to be quiet and still and experience the greatness of all that there is, with your mind and senses. This allows your consciousness to fly free and unite with the many heavenly souls who come to sing and praise the great Creator of all our universal dimensions. We Angels of light and love unite with groups of other Angels at every opportunity, for as we come together in groups, we share out light and energy and are energized anew. This enables us to carry on with our work, which is closely aligned to the human conditions upon the denser dimension of earth.*

We bring light to you so your denseness may become less concentrated and the earthly vibration may be lightened and become refined, so that the two worlds may draw closer together as the vibrations of each become more harmonious with each other. We use our influence by adjusting the energies around you so that you may respond accordingly. This enables us to steer you in the direction of your thoughts so that the physical operations open easily before you. This way you are sometimes surprised how easy it is to accomplish some things when the need has arisen to make changes.

It is because of your faith that the benefits of working closely with you, enables much adversity of physical matters to be removed or repositioned, so making your pathway clear and straight.

You might like to think of Angel help as having another domestic helper in your household, who will turn their hand to any task that is required, and make the general living life so much easier and lighter. We are here to serve in the best way possible and will always respond to the loving heart who dedicates their life and living to the help and healing of others.

Even Angels cannot help some humans because of their inability to activate their sensitive channel. This is when we use others upon the physical dimension, to act and provide help where it is needed, and where we cannot influence directly on a sympathetic wavelength. We often use a willing third party, to bring about the fulfilment of a personal wish, to prove that personal thoughts and prayers have been answered. This may be by actions or words or even by the written word in publications. In addition we have used the media of your radio and television to superimpose images, words and thoughts so recipients can receive our influence.

Mostly we use subtler means to influence and cajole as this is more beneficial, as the human believes it is their own mind which has brought the knowledge and information to light, so enabling a programme of movement, where previously there had been an impasse. We, who associate with the White Brotherhood, have knowledge of the human mindset, so we are able to use some aspects of the psychology of the senses, to assist in specific areas of concern. We may not be in a physical form as you perceive it, but we often stand beside you to whisper in your ear, nudge your auric emanations and hug you when our influence has been noted.

There is so much co-operation that spirit can give to any human being, who is willing to open their heart and mind to us. We want you to be grounded in your world so you can attain the best that each dimension can offer. This way your earthly life path will bring joy and happiness to the living of the present life and current existence.

God Bless you … Amen.

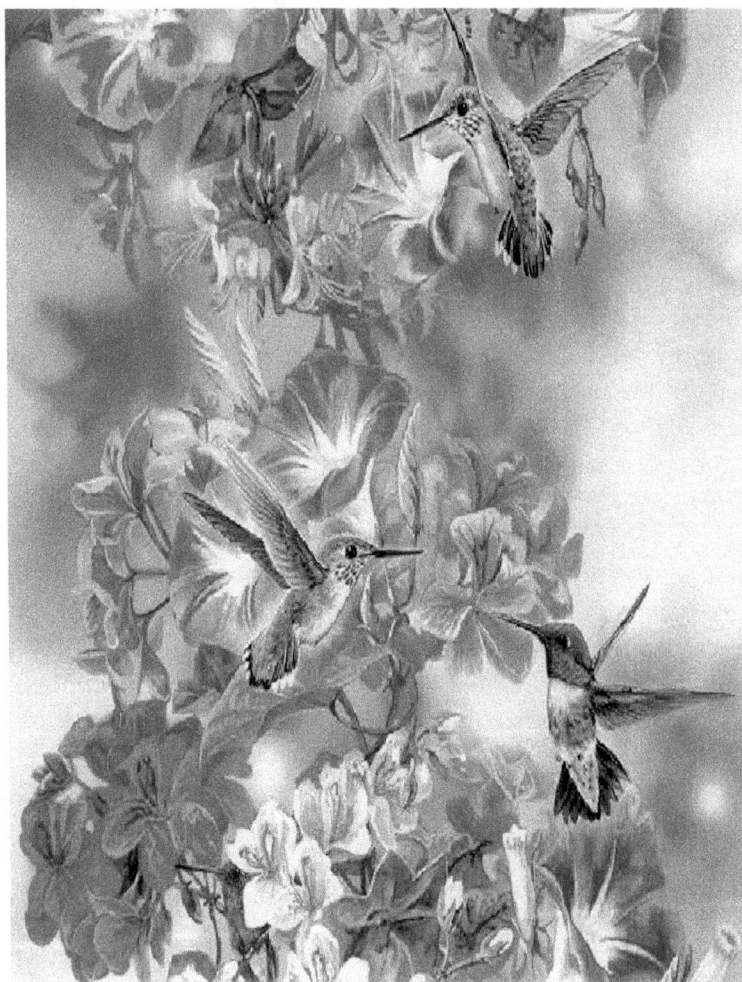

A Wonderful Sight.

Chapter 26

The House of Colour

On Saturday 23rd August 2008 I was asked to attend a meeting about a colour therapy. The therapy advocated was one of intuitive expression which lends itself to the personal clearing of emotional and physiological blockages of the self, by means of self administration.

This is accomplished by working through a particular colour which is identified from the source of some physical or emotional problem, to find out the underlying cause or causes which have been suppressed or hidden.

The workshops outlined, included the use of drama or theatre acting, to bring to the surface a demonstrated outward expression of the soul emanations showing negativity, so that renewal and intake of cleansing colour can then take place, to restore the balance and harmony of being.

What developed from this discourse was the explanation of colour as it impacts in our every day life. Billboards of adverts play upon our consciousness or subconscious minds, to evoke the subtle senses into action, so making the many human minds susceptible to the indulgence of the product being promoted. An example was a dark green background on a sweets menu, which relayed the message of being heavy and therefore was more often rejected as being too much to eat, on top of a main meal. After substituting a pale peach colour as a background to the advertised images, the sales from the sweets menu increased substantially, as the colour relayed a message of indulgence, so the human response was to treat oneself.

By studying the qualities of colour, the appropriate antidote colour can be administered. We know that bright primary colours stimulate children to learn, by attracting their attention through the five physical senses. We know also that aromas evoke strong emotions which can influence by attraction or repulsion. This happens in nature as a natural occurrence in the mating ritual and again in the survival mode. The moods we find ourselves experiencing may be the results of being immersed in a particular colour or aroma.

Experiments in Canada have recorded the affects of colour on people who have entered a colour room. In the red room it was found that people were individual in their approach and kept to themselves, while in the orange room the tendency was to fraternise with others and create relationships with interchange of speech and ideas taking place.

The yellow room produced people who were well on the way to expressing or putting ideas into action, as energies were dissipated this way and that, producing an emotional roll-a-coaster. By the time the green room was reached, the solace of quiet rest and balance was sought, to harmonise the frayed minds and emotions brought about by the immergence from the other room colours. Such are the affects of colour upon the individual. Such are the tools and materials for us to use to influence and command.

Where great strides are appearing or gathering force is in the beneficial affects of colour therapy on the healing of wounds and skin conditions. The affect of the blue ray of healing administered as pure light or coloured liquid, is seen in the fast recuperation of cell regeneration. There is apparatus today which defuses the colours of the spectrum to the requirements of a human's condition and responsive nature.

Many new age healers use crystals to activate these same colour amplifications to bring the healing energies into play. There are colour therapists who understand colour and the use of the different vibrations to bring about change within the body form. It is to these persons that the spot light should be turned, as it is in the application of colour that brings changes to all aspects of human lives and living.

The subdivisions of colour bring in the spectrum of hues and tones, depths and subtlety to change, defuse, enhance and enrich. The more the aspirant studies the aspects of colour, the more he finds to investigate.

The man who had come to provide this talk on colour has found an avenue of expertise, whereby he can use colour as a tool within the dramatic arts, releasing inner emotions and mental blockages within an individual and thereby clearing their negativity in a most positive and productive manner.

Those who have attended his workshops have enjoyed themselves and commented what an extraordinary experience it can be. It appears the intuition is employed and when directed, the individual can release their self diagnosed blockages and allow the transformation into wholesomeness to unfold.

We know that in the use of colour the benefits can be enormous. Those who aspire to fashions are driven by one colour or another. Those who are in the marketing profession use the tools of colour.

Those who are in the healing and health avenues use the colours for therapeutic purposes, as well as to enhance the beauty of all living things with the many displays of colour combinations, seen in nature or fashioned by man himself.

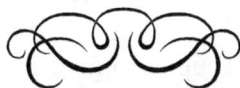

Chapter 27

Sensitive, Psychic or Medium
25/08/08 Broadcasting

I am your crusader come to talk with you again.

I come to tell you that the Brotherhood is assembling to ascertain the receptivity of the channels open to them.

A programme of direct communications is proposed whereby channels may approach the direct mind thoughts of individuals, or tap into the collective group thought projectors. Both methods will be used to find out the best method to relay information, as the time approaches when much influence is required, and much knowledge is sought, to meet the present needs of humans everywhere.

Spirit are moving closer to the earth planet as the veil between the two dimensions is very thin and it is like opaque glass that shows the shadows or outline of forms. If you stand close up to this barrier and blow upon it to shine a space, the opaqueness clears, to reveal a clear window. It is the intent or purpose that gives rise to the clearing fluid, so all will become visible and recognizable.

If you should find air blowing around your neck, know it is your Crusader who calls your attention. I may touch your ear and you may hear me whisper words into your mind. Know we are so near to you that we can touch you. Your attention is often elsewhere, so you do not register our nearness until you find the moments when you can quiet yourself. Then we can converse, as now, because you have heard our call and responded likewise.

Shortly you will be called upon to give a talk about how humans can become a channel for spirit.

First the sensitivity of the individual will require personal attention to determine the extent of their personal octave of operation. This is the spectrum they have developed as a result of earthly life and living and is what determines their range of sensitivity with regard to all things around them, and with those humans within their circumference of activity, with whom they relate and interact.

The greater the proficiency of operating this spectrum or octave becomes, will reveal the extent of the personal sensitivity of the individual. This will show by the awareness of nature and all natural things. It will also show the qualities and values of all living forms and the meaningful outcomes of expressions, which can demonstrate tangible truths of knowledge and understanding.

Such truths many bring to you a feeling of harmony and peace, which emanates from living trees and it may also be, that you experience the release of tension, on hearing the waves of water which ebbs and flows. To hear birds sing and receive upliftment of the tempers and to hear music and find yourself in a world of feelings, are all aspects of awareness due to your increasing sensitivity, that responds to the natural stimuli of energies around you. This may occur as a natural event or it can be a part of your daily life pattern. It may also occur when desired or induced to listen or play music, dance or meditate.

Certain sounds will evoke certain emotions, as will the aromas of perfumes. The natural perfumes are found in your gardens and countryside. The flowers, shrubs, bushes and composts have their own unique aromatic identification. Animals rely upon their sensitivity and you call it their instinct, as it is an inbuilt recognizable aspect of the animal nature or natural expression.

The next stage of instinct is intuition. This is a feeling or knowing that cannot be quantified and may be difficult to explain, for you are receiving impulses from the energy fields of others and the environment around you. Hence you know without knowing why. It is a part of your developing psyche or your psychic perceptions to know instinctively how someone else feels, thinks, reasons and acts as they do. You may even be able to predict their next move when recognising the probability note coming from their energy field, which emanates from their physical formation.

From your energy scan you can read and discern.

To activate the psychic mechanism, the lower triad of energy centres is employed. First the base centre at the bottom of the spine which shows itself as the colour red in a swirl of magnetic energy. This is used to provide raw energy to the form and to provide grounding. It gives grounding to the physical form to consolidate its attachment to the earth level of existence. This is a very powerful centre, as it provides the basis of form energy to activate all things physical and material, including the energies which interact upon you, on the earthly plane.

Second is the orange centre of the sacral area which provides the creative responses and brings this into being, by encouraging the relationships between the polarities of form. The vital signs are activated and animation occurs, so that the form may interact and exchange vitality with every action, sound, thought or imagining, so that the creative spark may ignite, to produce creation itself.

Thirdly at the solar plexus we find the centre of feelings that brings a qualitative additive to the vital form. This centre around the middle section of the torso is known as the sunshine centre for it can shine like a miniature sun. The five senses of the human vehicle allow it to move, sense, and experience this unique world of earthly vibrations.

Here we may indulge the senses and soak up the colourful vibrations that occur around and all about, in ever larger swirls of energy formations, that create the waves of movement to shape the NOW into forward progression.

The psychic operative uses these energy centres to scan for information which is held within the energy auric field of the human form, and in registering this wealth of information can relate to another human, their state of being and the circumstances that make up the present NOW.

The medium who acts as a channel for spirit communication may well employ the psychic and sensitive vehicles when undertaking a reading for a human who has come in need. Much that the human will require in order to be helped and healed needs to come from the level or levels that appertain to them and their need. The human being is made up of Physical, Emotional, Mental and Spiritual vehicles as part of his total makeup. All aspects of human nature must be balanced to enable a complete welfare of being.

Hence a medium will relay details of a loved one in spirit, to bring evidence of life continuance and details from them, to provide a communicative channel between the two worlds. This may heal the spiritual body for it may need reassurance that only a loved one can give. The mental vehicle may also be in need and once the contact has been made with the spirit loved one, the ripple of light will flow downwards to ease any mind and emotional turmoil.

The medium may be called upon to provide practical advice, so the employment of the psychic and sensitive aspects of being may be used, to give a clearer picture on how help may be best given or provided in the material and physical world. You may ask how the medium is able to make contact with spirit friends. This is a channel that all humans have to a greater or lesser degree.

To contact the spirit realms, the connection must first be established in a positive and factual manner. The mechanism needs to be tested and verified just like any energy or electronic wavelength service. By reaching into your heart or by reaching up to the stars, the realm of love and light can be accessed.

This employs the upper triad of energy centres being the Heart, Throat and Third Eye centre often referred to as the sixth sense.

Clairvoyance is clear seeing which is accomplished by using the third eye or inner sight centre, and many mediums use this method of communication in the first instance. Clairaudience is clear hearing and this faculty is use to receive names, words and dialogue without images. Clairsentience is clear inward knowing, where the inner hearing and knowing takes place.

In addition the heart centre provides the energy that reflects the communicator's emotional content so that the throat centre can verbalise these relayed impulses as communications that impress the mediums enhanced senses. The medium recognises these impressions as outside influences and can then relay the loving messages accordingly.

A programme of tuition will enhance any natural gifts to enable the blooming of the communicative channel in such a way that it becomes acceptable to the arena of operations upon earth. Since communication on the earth planet is now worldwide, many mediums are travelling internationally. Certain standards of operating channels are promoted as the acceptable general format.

As you may know, when spirit needs to get a message across as a matter of urgency, it may employ avenues from surprising sources. If a need is special, then special attention is employed where other avenues are used so spirit need to be creative in their approach, where it is appropriate and necessary.

This does not negate the value of a professional hardworking medium whose work of channelling takes personal priority. We rely on the work these humans generate, for great is their output and contribution to the human race and spirit. In recent times the spiritual hierarchy have drawn nearer to the earth planet than ever before, so the ordinary human may indeed connect to this spiritual level for help, assistance and enlightenment, by communicating direct.

It is in all cases of being, that the greater awareness is sought, for when you reach the conscious level of another dimensional existence, you then know that your spirit is universal and that you as a soul being, will have life everlasting if this is your wish and desire, as it is your rightful inheritance.

We here in the spiritual realms, ask the many humans to work in service for the Lord of Love and Light, so that the paradise of Earth may become the living reality, to bring the realisation of spirit expression at its highest, into the physical manifested world of earth, so creating the God-Man in the glory and beauty of our heavenly father.

Then the magnificence of the lighted illuminations will be seen as the presence of the **Great Omnipotent Deity** as our Universal Creator reveals his being and essence to us. This revelation is awaited by all who exist in the created dimensions of existence, so it is up to all of us from the universal dimensions of living, to establish the lines of communication from spirit, via spirit, to spirit.

In the knowing and acceptance of truth, we may unite in the oneness and wholeness of our divine source, to experience celestial glory and wonderment.

God Bless you.

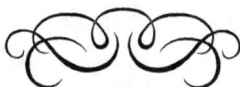

Chapter 28

The Hard of Hearing Club,
Cinderford. Gloucestershire.
26/08/08

I was visiting my father aged 87 for a week in August and on the Tuesday was invited to the Hard of Hearing Club at Cinderford in the Forest of Dean to listen to their monthly speaker.

A lady who runs the Coleford Hard of Hearing Club was the guest speaker and her name was Cath Hopkins. She came to speak about her life and how she has come to be a qualified Lip Reading Teacher. Her recent qualification has enabled her to offer lip reading lessons for the hard of hearing and deaf people in the Forest of Dean. The autumn course 2008 in Coleford is offered to hearing impaired people and deaf people in addition to the Hard of Hearing Club which she also runs to this present day.

Cath began by telling us about her early childhood. She had grown up with a hearing disability but this was not officially diagnosed until adulthood. She remembers the frustration of playing Chinese whispers at school and her friends becoming increasingly annoyed with her, because she couldn't carry the messages.

They thought she was stupid but in fact she was very bright and did well with exams. Her family were very musical so it was not unsurprising that she loved all things musical and aspired to become a music teacher. Throughout her schooling she overcame her disability by compensating or pretending when she could not hear.

It appears she could not hear the higher decibels of sounds so could not hear the birds sing or hear the whispers from her school friends. She made up for this lack by pretending, so she was able to go about ordinary life and living without much notice or attention by others, as to anything being wrong. When playing the recorder she could hear the lower notes but lost audibility at the top octave. She was in the orchestra as she had some talent, so she managed by blowing gently so as to make less noise, and that way no one noticed her deficiency.

Things came to a head when she was eighteen year old. She had earned a place at college and in those days you had to have a medical. She was able to pass the medical for her entrance to college by saying she could hear the ticking of a watch when in fact she could not. No one checked this, so off she went to college to become qualified.

She did in fact qualify as a music teacher and spent 20 years at local schools teaching the children musical instruments and singing. During this time she continued to compensate her hearing loss in various ways and asked her students to listen to each other to verify the top octaves of sound, which she could only register as vibrations. It may have been because of this that her groups all did well and were highly regarded.

However her hearing deteriorated and the stress of compensating by looking straight at people to lip read and then write up notes afterwards took its toll. A colleague told her she was singing flat when hitting the high notes and this brought it all to a head, as her health became affected by all the stress. She was devastated when she had to retire from teaching at age 41 years.

By this time she was becoming profoundly deaf so she attended the local lip reading classes to assist her communications. She admitted that she became very depressed as the silent world engulfed her.

Although many new friends were made by attending class, Cath wanted something more to do. One class teacher suggested she became a lip reading teacher but she could not afford the fees and the local job centre would not fund the course, as it did not meet the criteria for their funding. Additionally, the courses were only offered in London or Birmingham and required residency during the weeks at the college.

In the case of Birmingham, the course was run in six week blocks and the London courses were run alternate weeks. At the time, both these courses were beyond her means. She could not cope with being away from home and was unable to communicate effectively without some backup or support.

The idea was shelved so Cath looked around for something else to do. The local college of Higher Education ran evening courses and a pottery course appealed to her. First, she needed to meet with the tutor to see if he was willing to take her on as a student. The attraction to the pottery course was because it was creative but did not involve much listening, as it required a practical approach and application with the hands.

Cath arranged to meet the tutor before committing herself to this course to see if they would be able to work together. The tutor had not taught a deaf person before, but was willing to take Cath as a student, when she explained that he would have to talk to her face to face so she could lip read. She would require him also to show her how to do things, instead of just instructing her verbally.

The course went well – but not without its funny moments. Often Cath would be so absorbed by her tasks that when she looked up, she found herself all alone. The class had been asked to look at some technique or operation and had moved to one corner of the room to observe. Someone had forgotten to tap Cath on the shoulder.

No one meant to exclude Cath, it just didn't occur to hearing people that Cath needed that extra help with coping with every day events. Cath took to pottery in a very creative way and began producing some worthy items. It became her artistic outlet and soon Cath was displaying her creations and finding people wanted to buy her pieces.

An exhibition at the local tourist shop really took off and she continues to supply to them to this day. This activity provided some needy pocket money. Because she had made so many friends who were deaf or hard of hearing, she started the Coleford branch of the Hard of Hearing Club, so the Coleford residents didn't have to travel to Cinderford anymore.

The thought of becoming a lip reading teacher was still at the back of Caths mind. As the pottery became sought after, and Cath continued to exhibit her crafts, the pocket money became a small but steady flow to augment her income. When attending one of her hospital checkups she noticed an advert for people to train to become lip reading teachers. The contact given on the advert was someone Cath knew from another hospital she had attended, when going for tests to assess if she was suitable for a cochlear implant.

This operation had been discussed for some years but Cath had put it off, as she was doing OK with her lip reading and was able to cope. Suddenly it became clear that this operation would give her some advantage and take her away from the enclosed silent world that too often overcame her senses.

Because of her ability to lip read and now having more confidence due to the success of her pottery artistic displays, she determined that she would have the operation and duly underwent this four hour surgery in 2004. It took nearly a year for her to recover and gain all the advantages this implant offered, and for the first time in her life, she was able to hear the birds sing and identify the swish of closing curtains.

Cath talked in wonder as she described these new sounds but admitted that while she can now recognise these sounds, she doesn't have any memories of such things, as would be the case in a person who went from full hearing to becoming deaf.

So today Cath maintains that while she can hear the birds sing, they may not be the exact same sounds you or I hear, as hearing persons. She has no clear reference points to draw upon, so the sounds she accepts as birdsong may not be quite the same.

When Cath contacted the lady who was listed on the advert for the Lip Reading course, an interview was arranged. The governing trust duly offered to pay her tuition, although she would have to pay for her accommodation while attending the college. Cath chose the London College which ran the course on alternate weeks. This allowed her to stay with a niece who lived near by.

Cath had some amusing times while attending the University Hospital where the course was taking place. Travelling on the underground was a new experience. She realised that she would not have been able to cope, if she had not had her cochlear implant, as the noise and sounds of London life was something she had never encountered before.

Her course started in 2006 and Cath grew in confidence. Today, after reaching the age of retirement she is a qualified lip reading Teacher and runs the Hard of Hearing Group in Coleford as well as offering the new lip reading course starting September 2008.

The road back to teaching has taken her twenty years and demanded many changes in her life and in the living experience. With determination and fortitude propelling her forward she now finds many people gravitate towards her for help and assistance.

This is because she has been through the testing times and has not only the ability to teach a valuable subject, but can relate her own experience to others, to encourage them also to move on with their life, and never give up while there are others ways to circumnavigate the problems at hand. Cath emanates a glow of light which is clearly visible. She is an inspiration to everyone around her.

Those attending her talk that evening were all moved by her story. One man stood up and personally thanked her. He said on behalf of everyone present, that he wished he had met her twenty years ago, as someone like her provided a lifeline to those whose disability overshadowed their daily life.

She gave hope and a clear view that life doesn't stop, but could be carried on in different ways, just as fulfilling as it would be for hearing people with no disabilities.

This moving experience of meeting such a person who could relate such an uplifting story from adversity to success, reveals to us all that the spirit within each of us can rise to heights unknown. When we are faced with a hurdle to overcome, when we hear of others who have achieved such high abilities, we recognise that the spirit within some humans, is indeed one to applaud.

Caths story provides an example of how a life takes many twists and turns to provide a variety of experiences that benefit the one life in so many ways, that we as individuals could not have imagined.

Not all things in life are willingly chosen, some are foisted upon us for reasons unknown, but if we can rise to the challenges life provides and overcome most of them, then we may reflect upon our successes and be well satisfied we had done our best and made the right choices in bringing to ourselves, the best that can be achieved from the opportunities that life presents.

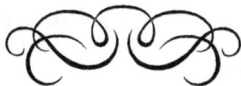

Chapter 29

Tuesday 09/09/08
Hitchin Healing Service.

Hu Lin Lo

I attended the healing service that evening and asked Steven to provide healing. I knew Steven had a Chinese Guide so I was not surprised to become aware of a Chinese gentleman from the world of spirit.

He told me his name was Hu Lin Lo which may have a different spelling to what I have used, as I can only relay the phonic sounds he gave me. He told me he was a doctor around the time of the 1800's when China was beginning to open up to the western world and missionaries were able to relay information back to the western countries via the trade routes.

I became aware of a large productive valley somewhere in central China. The peasant population was hard working, and while poor in worldly goods, were content and happy in their environment of simple pleasures and activities. The doctor was a central part of their community and well respected for his medical skills. In his status as a medical doctor he was regarded as just another of the community workers which made up the variety and scope of the many working people in this little world of county living.

The better off families were those who were engaged in trade, for that was the present growing industry or worth activity, so they could afford the brightly coloured fabrics and trinkets from the travelling merchants.

Most were poor famers living from their crops or produce with relatively little coinage. They could only gather coinage from anything surplus they could barter or trade.

Each household had its garden space where vegetables were grown. In addition the scrawny chickens and ducks roamed the nearby waterways which had been diverted from the main river to provide the irrigation for crops and rice fields.

In the village there was a communal wash pond where communal bathing and the washing of clothes took place. This was often a scene of delight as the children would involuntary help their mothers by diving into the pond on wash day, so this was how the communal washing of people came about.

Hu Lin Lo was a medical man who served this community in whatever capacity he could. Often he would be called to the labours of child bearing women and be asked to alleviate their pain and suffering. Many would pay what they could to be attended by him, as they knew he was an expert in the use of needles which he would vibrate at various sites on the body, to bring pain relief in childbirth and also bring relief for other ailments due to blockages of one sort or another.

In the bearing of children this therapeutic procedure was sought after, as the most effective method of assisting the natural birthing process. In addition this method of treatment would stall adverse bleeding and any complications could be dealt with most effectively there and then, while the patient was effectively wide awake and co-operative and free from experiencing pain.

Broken bones were often tricky cases to treat as the doctor had to rely on his clairvoyant capabilities if he needed to view the internal organs or tissue which had been displaced and affected by an injury. Hu Lin Lo was very adept at setting bones and prided himself on doing a good job. He had been a lad when his father broke a leg and the old medical man kept shaking his head when he was asked if he could set the bone and repair the damage.

Hu Lin Lo was just starting to learn the medical trade from another medical man who used the old methods along with the new methods of the day. Hu Lin Lo was a special student as he had demonstrated from a very young age that he had a gift or talent when dealing with medical matters relating to the human body, as he had an ability to carry out operations on people without using anything other than his hands.

He urged his mother to dismiss the medical man and took charge of his father's case. His father had sustained a complex fracture from a tree fall, when picking fruit. He first used his ability to entrance his father who fell into a swoon. He then went about setting the bone in a splint to keep the leg straight.

The bone had protruded from the skin so some tidying up of muscle and tissue was needed to affect a repair and some neat sewing of skin was required to make a good and pleasing job. Hu Lin Lo remembered to fashion a staff, so his father could lean his weight upon this stick to give him physical movement while the healing took place.

Hu Lin Lo's father recovered remarkable quickly and the word travelled some distance, about this talented young medic. This is why the doctor in adult life was always working as everyone in the local area wanted his attention.

Many people of the village and surrounding area were poor and so they paid in kind, keeping the doctors household filled with everyday necessities, so that the doctor would not worry about the mundane things of life, and could concentrate upon the peoples needs.

Many people volunteered to help the doctor by gathering herbs and making potions for the healing table, which was piled high with potions and plants that were often needed to alleviate some malaise.

At certain times the younger men would consume fermented rice water and suffer with digestive problems. This was usually treated by one of the potions that had been specially mixed for this purpose.

Some of the older men and women also had digestive problems and they were prescribed some soothing herbs to balance internal juices. Many of the older people suffered with aching joints due to the long hours spend in the fields planting, sowing and reaping. The poppy was known and a small supply kept, but respect was given for its uses, as it was known to have some devastating hallucinating effects, so it was kept for rare cases of need.

From time to time the children suffered from unexplained illnesses which manifested as fevers and rashes. One such child was the daughter of the chief trading man whose wife held office within the community and was known for her good works. The trading mans wife was a good looking woman with a homely approach, so she sent for Hu Lin Lo the moment her child became ill and feverish.

All that could be done was carried out, but still the child's fever raged and the life and soul hung in the balance. Hu Lin Lo was asked to perform the shamanistic rites as little more could be done for this child. The Gods were contacted. The Ancestors of old were contacted. The Great White Spirit was called, for the child was so dear to the family and was revered amongst the community as a special child, for she had been conceived late in life when all hope of having children had been abandoned and so had been considered a divine gift.

Our doctor became the shamanic medicine man and performed his ritual to evoke the spirits and healing powers. The village was silent as everyone prayed for the life of this child. In the early morning hours the fever broke and the soul of the child rested peacefully within the physical body of the recovering girl.

The life had been spared for a reason. The girl when grown was destined to enter into the healing profession and devote her life to the healing of others, so that the life force given to her could be transmitted to others as a special healing gift. This would endorse her special status and like our good Hu Lin Lo, people in this community and beyond, would come to revere the personage and work that was seen and carried out.

Hu Lin Lo now knew who his successor would be. He was pleased with the choice made, for he had often wondered how such a sensitive child had come to be the daughter of such material parents. He knew that his work would continue and that others would be brought into his life that would also wish to become holy healers.

This office of a community medic was more than the position of a general medical man, as it not only attended to the physical wellbeing of humans, but administered to the spirit or soul of the human being as well. It meant that the spiritual influences he was aware of, could continue to utilise a physical counterpart, to further the work of human betterment, welfare, progress and enlightenment.

The traders wife was influential and also wealthy and was well connected with the city dwellers over the mountains. Hu Lin Lo was happy that the spirits smiled upon him and his work. His mother and sisters who ran his household would eventually have a new mistress to govern them. He would take this child when grown to be his wife, so she could work with him, and all that he knew and owned would be hers as well. In sharing the work within the community, so much more could be accomplished. New and wonderful thoughts entered his mind so the future looked bright at the unfolding of events.

Now that many years have come and gone, Hu Lin Lo still influences those who come to his attention for medical assistance. His attachment to living humans is strong, so he uses his position in the spirit realms to show others how they may draw close to present day humans and assist in the present age whenever a need is highlighted.

Hu Lin Lo remembers the many years he spent in a close harmonious relationship with his lady wife who was his greatest helper and companion upon the earth. He remembers teaching her the old ways, by attuning to the stars in the heavens and many a night they would watch the night sky for movement and light.

He is now able to travel the celestial seas at will, but is always drawn back to the earth world where the many humans seek help, healing and enlightenment. Hu Lin Lo likes to show others how the energy patterns of the cosmos are reflected in the human body of physical form.

Now that more humans are coming to appreciate the more subtle bodies of energy, his work can extend to teach the relevance of attending to all the energy levels of the human form, which will require attention in some way and at some point, in the life span upon the earth planet.

The dense vibrations of earth are energy absorbing and the human form takes a battering when moving and interacting with the many other energy forms encountered. The natural world of earth also takes its due when the climate and living circumstances are continually changing, and the need for continual renewal is sought to enable the momentum of life to continue.

His influence is felt by the many light workers of the present age when they feel the necessity to act, speak or administer in certain ways when dealing with the healing and helping of others. He is particularly influential in impressing the thoughts to those that act the healers, and gives direction to the correct areas upon the body form for receiving the healing rays. This act assumes importance and relevance as his knowledge of energy flows comes into play. He knows how important it is to rejoin the connections of any frayed or broken alignments that affect the physical and etheric vehicles.

There are also times that his influence is felt when engaging in metaphysical endeavours, and since his knowledge and experience is extensive, his influence is given over a wide field of interest, from psychic surgery techniques to inspirational lectures on the healing of souls, as well as introducing the memories of old practices for present day needs and applications.

Hu Lin Lo loves Gods creations. He dedicates his existence to helping and serving humanity past and present.

He knows the benefits of bringing the earth world within the influence of heaven. He is one of many who are messages of God, and shines his light from within his own angelic being.

From his soul body form he directs the God energy vibration with cosmic deliverance, to all those he is able to contact.

Blessing to All………..A friend and fellow Light Worker.

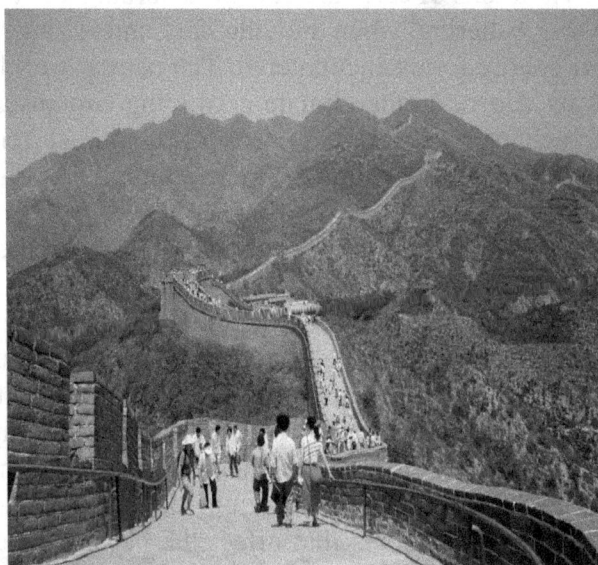

The long road to enlightenment

Chapter 30

Spirit Dialogue
Monday, September 15th 2008.

Dear One – Your crusader comes again in this quiet time just before sleep. Your mind is balanced as you have been reading about the Christ Light and its communications to your earth planet. It is true that the Christ, who you know as Jesus when upon the earth, has once again drawn near to humanity in thought and consciousness, for he dwells amongst us, the White Brethren and influences us also, so we may bring his messages of love and peace to the forefront of human minds and senses.

His ray of blue/white light is recognisable as your colour for healing, as it is this colour hue that has the greatest effect upon the body forms of humans and in particular to the regeneration of organic cell formations. This brings the physical form to its optimum efficiency and perfected display or structure and appearance. This blue/white light is most beneficial to the minds of mankind as it provides a healing balm to the emotions and mental vehicles, so enabling the energy rays to benefit at the physical material level.

The planet earth is often referred to as the blue planet with its vast seas and oceans, yet the whiteness of clouds which surround the globe, encase it and enfold it, like a fluffy soft blanket. Like a baby's blanket which is so light and fluffy, it secures the newborn in its warmth and softness.

Likewise the Christ love of the blue/white ray brings that aspect of God to humankind, so he may feel secure in that love and grow in the knowledge of that recognition of his soul or inner mind. This is his connection to this ray of healing love and through this blue/white ray, the awareness to the source, to that which is GOD can be found. At this time of ascension, the many changes and happenings in the earth world are causing waves of alarm amongst those who have set the material idols of wealth, power and control, ahead of peace, love and co-operation.

Many will be affected by the recent events within your financial organisations because the premise has been founded on shifting sands and much has been built on voids of nothingness instead of real creations of worth or need. Those, whose lives are affected by wider influences, may find their own personal circumstances undergo a major change and at these times the need for reassurance is great.

A new direction is sought and a new life pattern requires consideration. It is in the co-operation of the many that views and actions can be changed from selfishness to selflessness. Working for others to bring joy and happiness, knowledge and understanding, must be better and more beneficial than building castles in the air, for do you not seek personal satisfaction?

This can only be accomplished by giving to others and seeing the smiling faces and receiving their thanks for your administrations. Whatever field of endeavour you find to use, to demonstrate your knowledge and expertise, it is the education of Gods laws of rightful living that require spreading, so that those who are suffering may be helped. All humans must take responsibility for the calamities that befall, and seek to unite in groups, so you may pray and meditate to send the light beams out, for positive renewal.

You must ask for the help you need, by calling upon the angels and spirit guides. When you give your permission for spirit help, you will notice immediate action and see before you, how the energies are moved around and about to leave a pathway clear for you to travel.

As you build your own light and love vehicle, to allow your inner soul light to shine through your persona, you will emanate your own forward light and activate the energy forces, as the angels would have done, if you were not able to do this yourself. By enabling your own light body to be the directing force of light, you will have actuated your light body and truly realised your own angelic form, which shines as you truly are, as a light being of universal decent. Then you will realise that those in spirit and those upon the earth are exactly the same, only those upon the earth are garbed with an earth covering, making their physical contours and frame into the material body structure, which is 'YOU' here and now.

Your light form is the vehicle expression of the universe. It is through the light energy of the soul or inner being that the Christ consciousness can be met, and from which you can seek answers to all the questions you may still have unanswered. Know this, the blue/white ray is one of love wisdom and will always act to unite the physical to the etheric, the personality to the soul, the lower mind to the higher mind, and your spirit to the God source.

The blue/white ray aims to unite the polarities to bring the two opposites together and in this unity, the greater unity can be experienced, for you will have travelled back to source where enlightenment is found. So in your times of turmoil, times of great changes, attempt to quiet the mind and senses, so you may make contact with me and my friends who are grouped as the White Brotherhood, all working with the great light and love of the Christ consciousness to bring about the heavenly paradise upon the earth planet by sending the love and peace of Christ, to the hearts and minds of mankind and therefore bring about the transformation of the planet to its sanctified status.

To this goal, we work influencing where we can, teaching where we are able and sending love and healing upon this blue/white light that touches all creation, and transforms the material residue into positive growth, the dark into light, the unhappy into joy, and the earth into paradise.

God Bless You. Sleep Well..... Amen

Hugh de Lambert - Knights Templar.

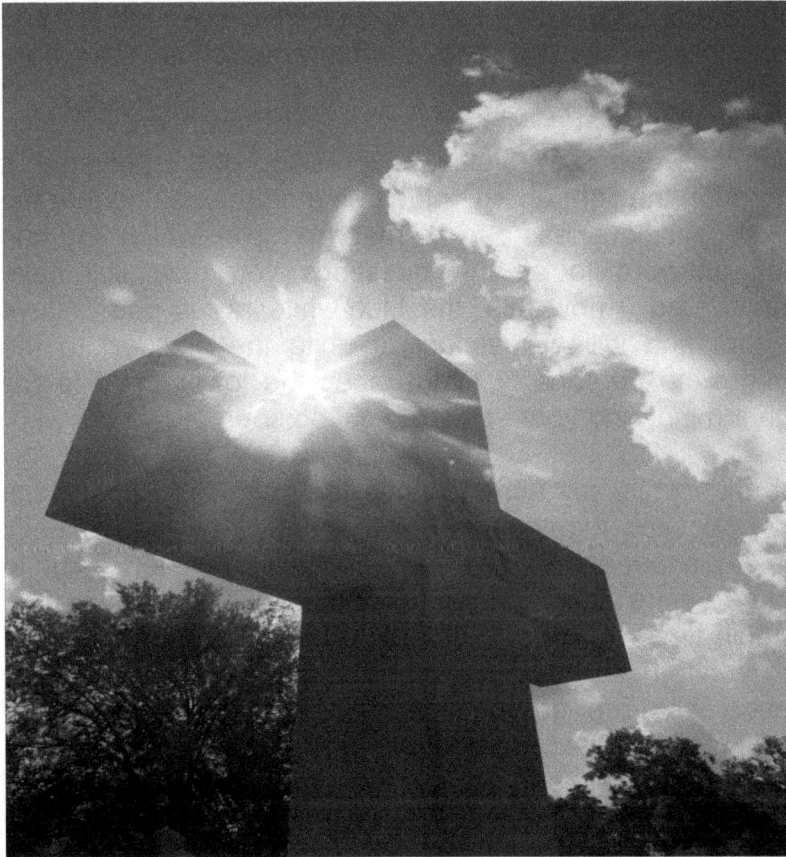

Christ's Light

Wednesday 17th September 2008.
Forest of Dean

We who draw near you come to speak as it is at this quiet time of evening that your mind is most receptive. You have found it much easier to accomplish your work when your mind is calm and free from fear. Such are the benefits of attuning to the higher dimensions where peace and tranquillity prevail.

In your countryside there are the signs of autumn beginning to show, as the leaves of trees are turning colour and there is a chill in the air when the sun is not shining overhead and the sky is covered with thick clouds.

You have found that the senior members of your race are very eager to enjoy the countryside and the more simple pleasures that abound and are within the budget of the many, so can be enjoyed. Many of the senior humans marvel at the pleasurable offerings of your world as they travel in vehicles around the locality of your present stay. Many have physical problems to endure but they take the opportunity to be among friends at every available event that unites them in the fraternity of friendship and companionship.

It is of interest to human adults to look at the young and see there are similarities, as the mindsets have reverted to self awareness and both relate in terms of their own self expression. The middle years of maturity are the years of learning and growing in understanding, so that the fruits of endeavours can be reaped in the summertime and harvest of your life experience. This way you cease to worry for you adopt an attitude of living in the moment, which is often joyous and beneficial to the days eventful happenings.

It is a lesson for all adult humans who stand between the child of youth and the maturity of senior citizenship. Just when you think you can relax and take life easy, you are propelled into activity by the demands of others who know that you are not ready to retire from previous duties and activities. Indeed, now is the time to adopt some new activities for the focus is on yourself to expand that which you already are.

Often a human will aspire to the creative arts and take up painting, drawing, writing, drama, music, dance, sport or yoga. It is also interesting to find that many who enter into the senior years are taking up the art of meditation. This not only allows the inner being to connect the soul or higher mind, it also brings benefits to the physical self by balancing those energies within the auric energy fields, to provide the best optimum harmony of health and physical operation. You may see the effects that meditation brings in those senior humans that glow with inner knowing, for they have made contact with the Christ consciousness and cannot help but smile to everyone, and transmit their happiness and joy at realising the wonderful truths hidden deep within the hearts of every human being.

Wednesday evening 17th September 2008

With the clock ticking you can see in front of your eyes the events taking place that have been predicted for your end times. When the house of cards falls, it does so rapidly and with great aplomb. These are the indicators of the great changes within society and countries that will change the world affairs and bring a greater co-operation between opposing fractions, as the residue becomes apparent, that no one person or country can live in isolation.

All must inter-relate and are dependant upon their brothers and sisters, as well as other countries for continual good fortune and benefit. Humble yourself to ask for help and see what responses are given. Look to your creator for your source of upliftment and courage and relish the contact with those of your friends in spirit who draw near at this time. Rise above the fear generated by the warmongers and those who feed upon the sorrows of others.

Shine your light of reason upon all those who need help and healing, to come to terms with their life circumstances.

It is often difficult to undertake life lessons when you may not consciously know why you are experiencing certain events or conditions. You only know you feel discomfort and pain. It is at these times that you question the finer truths upon which you base your life and when confronting life issues, you may decide to make changes that otherwise you would not have considered if you had been given other or different conditions prevailing.

It may be that you have been looking outward for prestige and wealth and need instead to look within to refine your inner light body, so that you may be able to give expression to your soul light and show to others, that your lighted vehicle of expression is poised in harmony and balanced peace.

This is depicted and shown as a strong lighted persona, full of confidence and surety and emanating a presence of magnetic vibrations that others may feel or recognise. Your light vehicle will be vibrating at a high frequency so that it attracts others of sympathetic notation, to your area of activity.

Many humans will then ask about truths, for if material or physical life is less meaningful, the void needs to be filled with knowledge and light, to bring you into the realms of awareness that you are now operating as a cosmic being. Your light vehicle can be seen and is registered upon both the physical and etheric levels of existence and manifestation.

Soon the spiritual beings of light will be able to show themselves upon the physical plane and likewise you will be able to visible show yourself to the etheric dimension. It is very exciting for many of us can then sit down together and relate to each other in more personal terms and much knowledge can then be exchanged with closer contact.

Thursday 18th September 2008

The waters of the river are swollen and high, and the greater force can be seen in the powerful surges of water through the channels open and unimpeded, to connect to the great seas or oceans of your world. The dramas of events are mirrored in humanity when fractions are motivated into action and move together like a stream or river trying to become part of that greater unity, which is represented by the great seas and oceans.

The need to amalgamate is strong within the make up of human personalities. It is an inner need that gives rise to the many extensive pursuits and relationships that occur within the living of earthly existence. A human being enters the world alone and exits the world alone. Yet during the life stay, there is a need to amalgamate with others, creating relationships and networking human influence. Always there is a striving to bring about a cohesiveness to unity, as unknowingly, man finds a distant longing to seek his heritage.

How many times does a man ask 'where did I come from and where am I going'. This age old question arises frequently from many souls all seeking answers from the living life. Be still and listen to the rushing water, for it will tell you its story. It is the stream of life whose origins are from the beginnings of creation, from the source of all things, that God creator, the universal deity whose mind and intentions brought creation into manifested glory, and whose presence is felt in the beauty and magnificence of all nature and its creations.

The God presence can be seen, within, without and around the earth planet, in the flow of the waters eternal movement. With the water and contained within its energy power, flows the vibrations of life, of light giving properties to enable the creative forces to amalgamate into form structures.

This creates life within itself, suspended within the waters, as all manifestations of the universe is suspended within the celestial seas which is part of the divine body of Gods form and presence.

Humans are constructed in his likeness, so if you look how you are made, you are able to understand that many parts make up a whole, and until those parts all beat in harmony, the best that there is, cannot bloom, for all has to beat as one, to experience the oneness of the greater being. This is why when you go into yourself, through meditation, you can rise above the physical form body and allow your spirit or soul to connect with the universal spheres and so connect with others who would like to join with you on your journey of discovery to the source of all things.

Your mind and emotions are clearly linked, so as you are able to free the mind and experience 'to be' so your emotional vehicle stands free, to express the being of self 'the ID or I'. Then you will be able to tap into the universal mind banks, which contain the knowledge for each existence.

Now you know why the saying of 'Be as a child' is meaningful. Learning begins again and as a child has no former concepts to colour its mindset, your being likewise, will benefit with little knowledge or no knowledge of universal matters, so you can see clearly and accept new concepts as they are given. To exercise your cosmic life suit is truly a marvel for the possibilities are endless. As a young child has to learn to walk, you too have to learn to manoeuvre by using your thoughts in a positive manner to focus upon your intent. Movement then follows thought power.

Once accomplished, the eager soul then wishes to travel extensively to see the sights, just as a child grows to adulthood and wishes to experience all things both at home and abroad. Like your many countries and climates the heavens are similarly endowed for as above so below.

Saturday 20th September 2008

The White Brotherhood are mobilising their forces by connecting the lines of light to those humans who are part of the ashram of souls that interconnect with the material life, to join it to the spiritual dimensions.

Many of the White Brotherhood have lived earthly lives and have influenced earthly living by their presence in personality, to leave to posterity a record of their life contributions upon the earth planet.

Many times incarnations have taken place to bring humanity some aspect of forward knowledge and to bring human understanding a step further in its overall accumulation of understandable truths.

In the present times a number of our operational ranks have again incarnated into the physical realm, to be present in the end times and so enable the alignment of the species to gain entrance into the forth dimensional awareness, by making that purposeful connection to spirit, via the soul or inner being, with the self direction of positive focus.

To consciously tune into the spirit airways is a great step forward. Not only does it show maturity of understanding, but shows a commitment to reuniting with the supreme source – our father **GOD** *– through that wonderful lighted presence of the Christ Consciousness. 'Through the Son is the Father reached'*

To aspire and achieve this state of elevation of the senses, is an accomplishment which is surprising, for so long have the masses ignored our ministrations that now, when we are viewing a positive response, our expectations are being surpassed, as many humans are now conversing with their higher state or mind where we can connect and relate much of import.

160

Today I contact you with much joy at the response of humankind which has surpassed all that we have hoped for. This does not mean that you can relax, for now that the momentum has begun, we must try to keep the tempo rolling and encourage greater speed and purpose in the near future. We hope to enable the forward propulsion of deliverance into the fifth dimensional awareness.

As you absorb the present cosmic ray vibrations which have activated the ascension process, you will find your fourth dimensional living conditions extremely interesting. Many more beings will present themselves and a truly colourful interchange will ensue.

We can see a time ahead when physical life is more settled and everyone is focused upon the self development awareness processes. This will bring greater clarity and understanding. Humans will live by right thinking, right relations towards others. Co-operation and welfare will be priorities and the land of earth will blossom anew.

Your paradise is already in blueprint.

Act now to make this your reality, so that you may benefit from its bounty and know that your children and children's offspring, will inherit a heavenly homeland in which to live and express their cosmic heritage upon this newly sanctified planet and world called Earth.

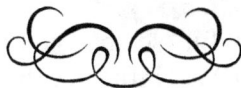

Chapter 31

Melanie Polley's Autumn Family Gathering 2008
Scarborough, Yorks UK.
12/10/08

Spirit dialogue:-

We the Cosmic Lords assemble at the high place outside of your world to bring about those lines of connections which enable the avenue to open for dialogue between us. We have brought you here again, to this special place to begin preparation on the construction of your re-fitted vehicle. The special equipment needs attuning within, that only specialists can accomplish, so we have employed those upon the physical world who will understand our requirements.

Your present tutors may give you different explanations with regard to fine-tuning your apparatus, but we will use this opportunity to bring about the wanted alterations that will allow the finer vibrations to be channelled through your vehicle of expression.

The present refit has given rise to new equipment being installed within the energy field of your physical vehicle, so that the width and breadth of your services can be activated to accomplish the best clarity and understanding possible. Because you are a human and constituted of flesh and bone which makes up your physical body, we have to fashion etheric counterparts to be incorporated within your aura or energy field, so when you operate the channels of connection, the amplification can become employed, and your broadcasts can reach a greater audience than otherwise would be the case.

Know we are ever watchful, so that you can take advantage of opportunities that arise. We influence to bring about the best advantages of energy and places and are thankful for your responses to bring our influence into material occurrence and success....................God Bless You

The Light of Purity.
13/10/08

Spirit dialogue:-

The portals open and again we can communicate. Dearest, we draw near so the energy of cosmic purity can be brought to the group, to ignite the souls attending this session of activity. In uniting together in this way, you are concentrating the light to such a degree that when sent with positive intent, it can be seen as a laser light beam rising into the cosmic regions of time and space to connect with the land of universal deliverance.

At this time it is important for enlightened humanity to pull together in thoughts, words and deed. The earth world is undergoing the repercussions of changes already occurred and now solidified within the heart of your planetary form. The light vibrations of purity are burning away debris of negativity, to bring cohesion amongst all things. Whether it is the kingdom of nature, or between human societies, or humans themselves, the changes affect everything in some way and unites one with the other.

When you are striped to your soul; light from your own being, the sun of yourself, shines forth to display your essence and reality – neighbour will call upon neighbour for one will rely upon another and separation will become something in the past. All is accomplished by the light vibrations which are being changed to a lighter, vibrant scintillation, so that the earth heart and soul may gain expression in its manifestation upon its outer adornment, to affect all those creatures existing upon its surface and beyond, into the earths atmosphere surrounding the globe and encompassing it within its ring-pass-not.

The planetary Lord is overseeing this process and is conscious of the necessary delicate operations needed, to bring about the planetary transformation. Bringing Gods glory to shine as a tangible reality within the material plane of expression is a goal of reality that has long been held. In the presence of such glory and abundance, all souls can shine more brightly and enter into the reality of multi-dimensional travel and existence. To witness such phenomenon makes the souls understanding take a huge leap of growth, so it may become, and express itself, as the universal or soul format of its original seed. A momentous delivery of a transformation, that happens rarely, but once in an age.

To the earth planet, this transformation process is a magnificent event, as the species of humankind is in its awakening state to reveal in the physical form, the spirit or soul aspects direct nature. To express this heavenly or divine attitude of being – physical form is to see a transformation most glorious. It is that which is only imagined from the stories of angels and heavenly beings of ancient heritage and origins of past legions. Truth of being will be revealed as the light from the cosmic sources connect with the inner light stream of your human being, so bringing about, that flowering and transformation from plant to bloom, in this most divine and pure revelation of your consciousness.

Higher Self and Consciousness.
13/10/08

Spirit dialogue:-
I am alive. I am alive which is more than can be said for some of those in front of me. I am alive because I can register the life energy that flows through my being. Can you register the light flow through your being? Most people are not aware of the greater awareness from what a human can now achieve. We learn from childhood to become aware by using our five senses of smell, touch, hearing, sight and taste. When we have attained adulthood and sometimes earlier, the human can begin to develop the super senses of their being, which will enable them to register their environment, within the earth world, in another manner or different way.

By enhancing physical hearing to clairaudience, by enhancing sight to clairvoyance, by enhancing the senses of smell, taste and touch to a higher level to evoke clairsentience the whole of expression known as man becomes acquainted with his etheric counterpart, that vehicle of energy known as your auric emanation or spiritual essence. It is here that the registration of subtler energies can be observed and viewed. Much that is visible within the etheric vehicles of the physical being can be seen working out in the physical body form of the individual man or woman.

To become aware of the energy flow within the physical body, you must first register or come to understand, how the etheric energy centres work and play, to influence the whole vehicle of human expression. To register if you are truly alive, is to become aware of both the physical and non-physical vehicles as they express the life flow, as seen or felt by your physical or non-physical sensing. You may feel the power flow by registering the coloured lights that show themselves in an etheric form when the centres of energy flow and connect to each other.

So when I say I am alive, it means I can see and organise the life flows in both the physical and non-physical vehicles, which makes up my person, so it can make it shine and glow and be seen by others as being all aglow. Someone who glows, will glow with the life light of our cosmic power source.

This comes from the Great Omnipotent Deity we call GOD. Once you have connected to this source of light and power, you will know for sure by your feelings and sensing that registers the maximum velocity of energy that is presently known, and can be felt and absorbed within a human form.

You will find yourself lit up to glow with a fluorescence amounting to the output of thousands of light bulbs from your earth world creation. Then you can say you are alive, for all will see it is so, from your light emitions.

.............................Your Light Being.

Operational Developments.
14/10/08

Spirit dialogue:-

Dearest, my presence will be known today as I draw close to you. This should not cause you any problems as I am often with you in your daily life, when you are engaged in spiritual activities, particularly healing and teaching.

My guise you can register as you have often been aware of me and know I bring a love essence that is all protective and fulfilling. Today we will explore the workings of your new mechanism which has been implanted to provide a greater amplification. If all works as it should do, you may find on the physical level a greater surge of love energy and all dealings with esoteric matter will be more readily recognised and you will know how to deal with the energy flows given.

We wish you to have a good experience as many would like to use your channel. We must make sure that the working parts are all in good working order and that you as the recipient are happy with the feelings that this work brings.

You know you are protected as the Crusader and I work together to bring the channel into operation, so that the Brotherhood members can have another outlet for their discourses. The Brotherhood are instrumental in providing the vanguard for those working and engaged with the ascension process. The Brotherhood specifically deal with mans understanding and attitudes, many of which need to change, to acknowledge and absorb the Christ light and energy, for the betterment of the human species.

This Christ energy is transforming and needs to be understood in detail, as you will encounter some troubled souls who have become tangled up and need unravelling, before the light can reach those parts of denseness to clear the debris from their beings. This is where the healing comes in, for healing is all about bringing the vehicle of expression to its optimum equilibrium and receptivity.

The soul needs to be brought to a point of balance within itself and its known heritage. The scales must be evenly balanced for the individual to move forward. You understand now why it is necessary to prepare first, before the functioning of your apparatus. Know, once this new channel is operational, a flood of information is likely to be transmitted. You will be surprised at what will be broadcast.

The finer the tuning made NOW, will have bearing on the quality of broadcasts, as like your radio receivers, the station needs to be connected on a strong vibration, as otherwise the receptor will crackle and pop as the energy vibrations waver this way and that. We have constructed a tall aerial transmitter to aid your broadcasts, for we are confident all will be as we envisage, as like all new innovations, there may be some added advantages that have yet to be discovered. Enjoy today. Enjoy the energy vibrations sent your way. Come to recognise the different flows and working mechanics of the altered state of consciousness, so you will be able to help others and be instrumental in opening other channels alongside your own.....your Nun Guide.

Morning Meditation –
Connecting to Mother Earth.
14/10/08

In being asked to connect to mother earth, I became aware of each spirit centred within the trees and vegetation upon the surface of our planet. They would not let me go into the earth as it was made clear that they were there to support me as grounding; by grounding the energy to propel me upon the spiritual path which was displayed in front of me. It was straight but had a very deep steep dip before climbing a hill which was where my vision stopped.

As I began to walk upon this roadway, the vegetation at the sides of the roadway came to life. Earth spirits suddenly appeared and came to join the procession gathering behind me, making sure that the foundations and support from the earth vibrations were following behind, to anchor me while I soared ahead.

I became aware of the Red Indian colour wheel which depicts the zodiac of existence to give understanding of life continuance. My new view of this colour wheel was given as a cone with indented sides which seemed so unsymmetrical. It made me think of a pawn shape on a chess board. Each segment on the colour reel is a colour stream and I was shown that the bands or lines of horizontal levels denoted the levels of each existence, and reminded me of latitude lines. These levels all narrowed in circumference as they rose to the godhead at the dome or apex of this apparition. The bubble at the top was just like the pawns you use for a game of chess or draughts.

Most humans know about the human level and those who aspire to higher levels will understand that the forth dimensional consciousness is responsible for depicting the symbol of the cross with a circle at its centre, to reveal the point of evolvement of the human development for most intelligent human beings. On the zodiac colour cone the light pathways to the summit are at each edge of a coloured section, and these are the traditional avenues of transition for incoming and outgoing soul emanations. Human consciousness has given rise to a new pathway in mid section of the colour segment along the meridian lines or matrix lines, which act as the longitudinal lines of the web of interconnectivity.

This web connects all other dimensions with the universal existence. Hence the meaning and understanding of 'We are all as one'. This super light roadway, for that is what it has become, is wider than a pathway in your understanding and is generating much interest from both sides of visible incarnation. The light beings are visiting the human souls which can respond to the finer vibrations and are encouraging visits into the spiritual dimensions. These visits bring greater understanding to many humans and the glow of the Christ energy is being absorbed.

The construction of this intergalactic highway is being constructed from love energy as the Christ wishes to bring home all human souls within this matrix and the best way to do this is to construct a vehicle which will allow the mass integration of a species, with swift precision and accuracy, so that the original plan will work out, although the road to this manifested ascendancy has had many twists and turns.

Always the supreme intelligence has held fast, to **hold with the light**, the most densest of his creations, believing that the love energy will transform, will revitalise, will create that which was the masters intent. In doing so, the human race, by their own volition will be endowed with Gods attributes, for he fashioned humans in his likeness and it is into the faces of divine emanations that the creator wishes to view, when the eyes of the human soul mirrors the universe, then will the soul know of its homecoming.

The human realisation of existence will move to the collective mind of GOD and become a part of his being in the true sense. This is what is meant in becoming a God. All have a pathway to follow, all have the dream, all have the pull towards Gods love and light, so follow this vibration and you will find your pathway home. The light pathway nearing construction upon the colour segment is shown or viewed as the cross, at the point of intersection being the node at which humankind exists. The pathway of light can be traversed while in the physical life, for the two worlds are nearing and will become as one. Heaven and Earth will combine and everything of energy form will become visible and reveal themselves. You will view your status to others in different dimensions.

Best behaviour, best thoughts and best outlook is called for, as we do not want to disappointed others nor do we want to disappoint ourselves.

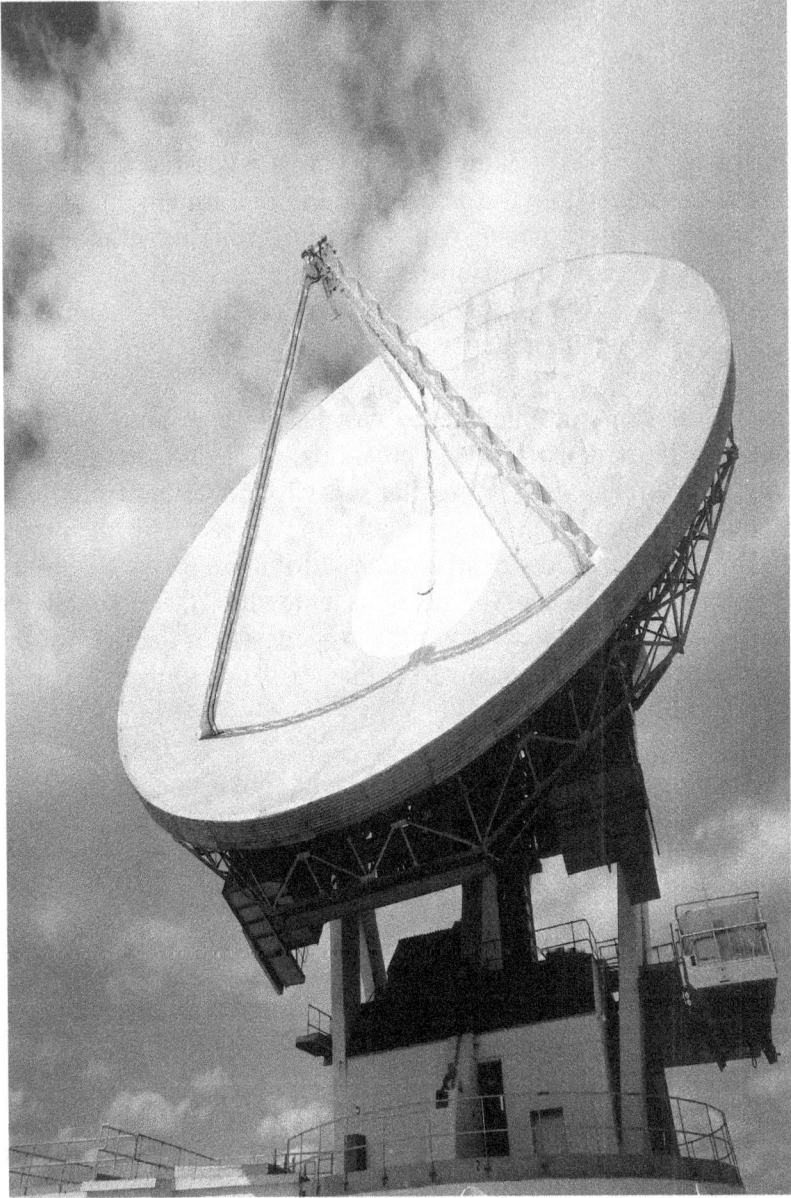

Communications

Moon Star
14/10/08

Spirit dialogue:-
The moon shines an eerie light upon the stream and casts a shadowy reflection of the moon upon the water. The moon is a planetary disc that reflects the suns rays even though the sun does not have direct access to that which it illuminates. The moon is reflective in all its attributes as it looks past the outer covering to look into and reflect the meanings or interpretations. All energy carries values and colours within its flows of life power.

A picture is a reflection of a real manifestation or it can be a reflection from inner sights and feelings. Both tell stories that can educate and inform. Much is learnt by recording experiences both inwardly and outwardly so that others who undergo a similar occurrence can understand the meanings more easily. So much beauty can be relayed by reflective glory. Much that is seen is relayed via a mediumistic channel in the reflections of images of different times, places, and dimensions like a movie, a run of images can make up a story and understandings can be achieved.

-------------------- o--------------------

'In my life I was Moon Star daughter of the chief of our group of Indians. We lived on land which you know as Canada within distance of great mountains and forests. This was a fertile land and we lived in a valley enclosed by mountains where we saw the seasons come and go. Wintertime was cold with snow and ice but the stream that ran through our valley kept flowing, even when the thickest snows covered the land. The best fishing was in the lake which was lower down from our valley home, where the forest animals congregated.

This area was safe, for visits from neighbouring groups tended to be made at the lakeside in spring and autumn time where exchange of goods and produce was made.

The spring gathering was particularly welcomed as renewal of basic items was always sought. During the winter months the women would make garments for summer and winter, headgear and moccasins, water and holding bags, tent panels, blankets and skins, as well as useful items of needles to sow, hand tools, plates and bowls.

Many of these articles were embroidered or painted with decoration to show the tribe or group which identified the source peoples from which it came. I was always enlisted to design the patterns for paintings or drawings on the tepee panels and also for the decoration on all the garments worn for display or ceremonial purposes.

We were fortunate for the area of our valley afforded us with the special coloured earth dust which in the spring months could be gathered and made into the paints used to colour the drawings. In addition the men would use these paints for the ceremonial occasions of ancestral gatherings when the local family groups would gather in celebration of nature's solstice.

I was often inspired by nature's patterns in each season as well as the mountain, stream and forest spirit manifestations, which showed different aspects of their nature according to the time of year. The animals also brought inspiration as much of our culture was associated with the indigenous animals of our land. Many of our stories were based on the activities and behaviour of animals so our children would understand those that were friendly and those that were not.

I had four children which grew to adult years, three sons and one daughter. Another son and two daughters were laid to rest beneath the tall pines as they retuned to the great white spirit as infants during the time of the great freeze. My eldest son was Running Bear who was brave and showed little fear. He became a good hunter and leader of our peoples. My second son was Grey Fox who also was a good hunter and very agile, for he could climb the mountain side with ease to collect the medicinal herbs that grew upon the high rocks in the pure air. He became knowledgeable about such herbs and was considered a grand shamanic healer. My third son was Red Wolf who was cunning and thoughtful when calculating his moves and became a great advisor to the nations.

My daughter Rainbow Aurora was the blessing of my life, for she shined with the colours of the rainbow and her goodness of nature was mirrored within her aura and could be seen reflecting the rainbow colours. She had the sight and ear of the Great White Spirit for many would come to seek her assistance when troubled in spirit and in life.....More of this life and my husband later.......

Morning Meditation.
15/10/08

Spirit dialogue:-

I come from a star system some distance from your own planet which is beyond your comprehension. You know me as a Cosmic Lord for I with others have responded to your light call from the large gathering of souls. We are considered Star people as we exist around the stars placed in the heavens.

We work with the energy and power for universal needs and oversee distant planets in their development of consciousness. It is interesting to find that when you earth people gather into groups to 'commune' and send out your vibrations, you evoke the cosmic laser lights into action, which are used to bring the cosmic beings nearer, as a call sign for help and healing on a planetary level.

In your case it is an invocation of celebration, that your consciousness has registered the ability to contact us, and in doing so, intelligence can be imparted between us. The old race of man who honoured the Great White Spirit was a developed group living on your planet, whose origins came from the star people and their planets. They came to the earth to ground the knowledge of their history and origins, to bring to subsequent generations of human beings, the understanding of universal wholeness and the respect for the Great White Spirit as it is shown in all the manifested glory of the earth planet. Your world is an experiment to see how far a human can travel and develop consciousness while housed within a dense physical form.

To know that a group can transcend the barriers and restrictions of the physical form and connect to the real world of energy formation and power is a marked development of the race. This brings us so much nearer together in mind relativity and marks the race as achieving its graduation into its cosmic heritage. We, who normally stand aloft, view, observe and send our thought power to the planetary beings of the universal spheres. We can communicate with individual minds if that mind is sufficiently robust, to reach out or shine the soul light to provide a beacon to us.

This you have done today and we find you surrounded by star people who live in the ethers. They are very excited and are celebrating this gathering of inter-dimensional interchange and greetings. It seems that the star people who inhabited your world long ago, are still watchful and waiting. They stand together to assist and guide the race, in the understanding of the great concepts of the continuing life.

The ways of spirit progression are complex, for many have Free Will and exercise this faculty to take them on journeys throughout the universal spheres. This has attracted other species of cosmic heritage, so now many humans have different entities as helpers - from far flung planets and systems. All are willing to help and bring knowledge to the earth people who are struggling to bring the earth planet back to its sanctified status amongst the central star configuration.

The planetary systems are like a large matrix, connected together by beams or lines of light energy. It is to this connection that the earth planet is nearing so it can connect to this centred matrix and join with the other evolved souls that have perfected a multidimensional mode of expansion. Spirit, Etheric and Physical. Know that the Cosmic Lords are watchful and are joyous at your activities to bring greater light and love into your world, and to its peoples. Know that the central source, that intelligence of all powerful knowing you call GOD, is well pleased and adds more power and light to your endeavours, by sending to us – The Cosmic Lords – a fine beam of pure power and love to say 'Thank-you' for your purposeful call.

We will speak again shortly – Four Cosmic Lords speaking as one.

Class Activities 15/10/08

Our class consisted of nine people including two Loraine's and two Jenny's. One of the Loraine's was asked to adjust the lights by switching the end lights on and the front lights off, in the main hall that we were using as a classroom. She tried a number of times and as she turned one set of lights off, they would come on again. This happened five times and in the end we all laughed as the thought occurred to us, that it could be Melissa a spirit child, who was a main guide of our tutor, who always likes to play games with the visitors attending these courses.

During class activities one member performed shamanic healing rites and another assisted in removing negativity from the energy forms of those present. We undertook various meditative exercises to bring our guides closer so a clearer connection could be established. I registered the presence of a Red Indian. He gave me a name of Grey Cloud but I could not register his presence other than a high energy field and no other words were forthcoming so I was not willing to say anything on such vague sensing. I was obviously wrong, as the tutor told me afterwards that he had told her I would not allow him to speak through me. This was a lesson for me to understand the mechanisms prevailing for the deliverance of a trance dialogue, so I should know next time the way of things.

Evening reconnection
15/10/08

I was transported to the higher realms to assemble with the Cosmic Lords. This was a healing of some import. A good number were assembled in a semi circle around the throne upon which a Lord was sitting. He directed his light upon us and as it travelled from one to another the physical body or covering vanished to reveal a lighted being of glowing proportions. As I looked at this, I realised we are all cosmic beings and exist in essence as energy forms of light, which can be fashioned to any race or planetary tribe, according to the prevailing directives and wishes of the Lord.

I also became aware that those assembled were not all from the earth planet, but this didn't seem to make any difference when being presented to the Lord. All were creatures of creation and beneath the outer covering all looked alike in their cosmic suits or light bodies. As this recognition occurred between those present, there was great laughter and delight. No longer was the air apprehensive with mystery, all was revealed in simplistic splendour.

All the light beings began to shine from their energy centres as the light of the Lord came upon them, as a spot light identifies the specific, each one of us was illuminated. Present souls revelled in the glory of this eventful understanding. The Lord was pleased that so many rejoiced, for he had a directive for each and every one. *'To put on the outer garments again and return to the planet of experience and choice'*. There was a lull and a pause while the magnitude of this request was absorbed.

It was explained that the mission to return to chosen worlds, was to take this knowledge to the many that have not seen, for blessed are those who would believe but have not born witness. For those who have received this revelation and knowing, the task of spreading Gods knowledge of love and light to all living creatures would be their task. We were told that when the planetary life was ended, we could all return to find our light shining even brighter and know that we had served the Lord well.

I became aware that the good Lord has sent many messengers to the earth planet and else where, to plant the seeds of knowledge and truth for others to know, so that the Lords lighted presence may manifest upon the planets of his creations, to provide a heavenly paradise for souls to reside for all infinity..

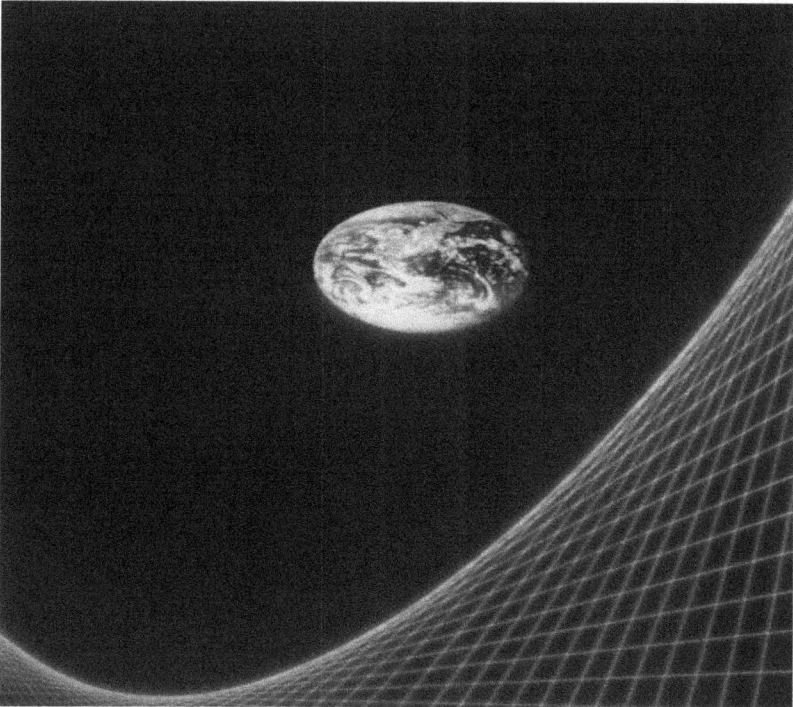

Planetary Dimensions

Morning Meditation.
16/10/08

Spirit dialogue:-

At morning break the air is crisp and the mind alert. This is when communications are clearer and easier as the airways have been purged of the debris of yesterday. We who stand apart to observe, are well pleased with the progress taken this week. The energies have been aligned and new connecting strands have been put in place.

This can only be accomplished by our light engineers who fashion our blue print with expertise and precision. The lines created this week are shinning with newness. All is ready for use and we are expecting some good results.

Individual humans do not always know the heritage they carry, for if they did the burden in the one life would be too great. This is why much previous knowledge gained from spirit soul existence is left behind when incarnating anew. A new child is a pure vessel to be filled with the physical life energy that takes the soul enclosed within on a journey of discovery through the physical five senses and then, as with all evolvement, the circle completes another round of experience and is taken on a higher level of the life spiral. This happens to a child when it reaches adulthood and again at senior initiation.

Therefore your twenty years or more are geared to take you to the consciousness of your soul journey in line with the fourth (being 20years *4 =80yrs) and fifth (20years *5=100yrs) dimensions.
Therefore your three score years and ten (70yrs) relate to the average level of attainment, which equates to reaching halfway upon the path to the fourth dimensional realisation.

Many are reaching this level beforehand and no longer have to wait for the passage of years. To those who live longer in the physical life do not take this as a signal that you have not developed sufficiently.

Many have moved to a level where they can teach the valuable knowledge of the mechanisms and workings of life energy forms and the correlation of Gods kingdoms of how they interlink with one another.

The human species is diverse in soul development and understanding. Some are becoming more in tune with the planetary being and an emergence of all things Shamanic is becoming known. This is a physical display of harnessing the power and healing vibrations that come from the planetary centre and is manifested in the kingdoms of nature.

From the mountain and earth spirits to the animal and plant divas, the flow of cosmic or spiritual radiation is mirrored within each creation to connect itself to the cosmic star creator. So, a human can look back and forward, up and down and see the circular flow of energy that connects him to the Great Omnipotent Deity 'GOD' which is focused and implanted within the manifested form, whether it be the planet itself, or the creatures of form residing upon the planets surface, or that which is contained in the planets atmosphere or ring-pass-not.

The sounds brought about by the animals and used by the souls of the star people, the Red Indian Nation were very strongly connected and used in their time of living upon the planet. Now, those who were strong with the shamanic force re-connect that power and knowledge as it can have great impact on the physical level of existence.

Those who wield the cosmic power for healing and live in the etheric worlds outside your planet draw close. The hierarchy of Ascended Masters are wise in their deliverance to send help and healing in what ever form is appropriate to those presently incarnate. When both power houses of Yin and Yang are employed, the balance is produced and where balance and harmony prevail, the light and love of Christ is centred and all is made well and whole again. This gives you much to think about and assimilate.

You may be aware that from the spirit above and below, the human levels are making themselves known. Mans heritage is to have dominion over the lower three kingdoms of nature, so as an earth cosmic being, Man as a species will develop his powers of controlling the energies. As above so below, man will himself manifest his goodness by bringing the balance and harmony to the living life.

This is the gift that the Great Omnipotent Deity has given to Mankind and explains the understanding that Man was created in Gods image. Man has the ability to bring peace and balance in the kingdoms of nature, the mineral kingdom, the vegetable kingdom, the animal kingdom. Man also has the ability to harmonise at the physical level, the emotional level and the mental level.

The pathway is clear so Man can ascend to his rightful place as a co-creator, to sit at the right hand of Christ, that supreme being that brought about the creative forces to manifest those kingdoms for man's control. Do you now understand that the group soul which is the human race is a Son of God, to govern his kingdoms of manifested glory, to the magnificence and wonder of all other creations. Man was given 'Free Will'.

It is this which has been a blessing and a curse, for in mans search, in mans journey to understand he has had to face many trials and tribulations. The soul needs to be tested.

The soul must stand strong, so that it can deal with every occurrence imaginable, to bring the energy power source to its balanced state and allow the realisation of all Gods love and light into the individualised component or cells that make up the species of manifested mankind.

God Bless You All.

Healing Session.
16/10/08

The healing service started with prayers and all spoke the names out loud of those who required healing at this time. Two beds were set up as healing tables and six chairs sited alternatively for spiritual healing.

My healing was with Sheila who quickly was guided to the area of my body that was recovering from recent major surgery. In addition I had been suffering from some digestive problems which were the reaction from the various energies employed during this week of activity. Hands found the appropriate parts and coolness was felt where heated areas had arisen.

I became aware of my guides who had been identified earlier in class. One that I was not familiar with, but for some time I have received their influence, not realising that recent pictures and experiences were brought to me via this gifted guide. I first registered my Nun and then became aware of Grey Cloud the Native American Indian who was recently introduced to me. He was particularly strong and agile as in an earlier life which I registered, and I recalled that I had been his wife Moon Star.

I was told to write about his life and in doing so would learn many truths. The knowledge gained would be of interest to many who are influenced by the star people and realisation on many levels would occur.

Another influence registered at this time was of an Egyptian. I have often been aware of this influence but have not yet seen a face or person from that period. I did become aware that I was wearing a tunic that came to above the knees and my legs seemed bare. I had some headgear to signify some status but I cannot recall anything else, just the knowledge that this influence was full of ancient knowledge of the life that was led and the esoteric knowledge of that time which was rapped up in myths and beliefs about the afterlife and the Sun God Ra.

I kept seeing the cross displayed as healing hands moved from one position to another. I registered my main meridian was being strengthened as this had been damaged by my recent surgery and I still need assistance to connect the lighted lines of the meridians to strengthen anew.

Last but not least the influence of shamanic practices was expressed to me. The attributes of animals known as the totem guides, were there to connect and give greater power to ground me and offer further understanding about those energies appertaining to the earth divas.

Again I was brought back to the Red Indian Star Nation, and their contribution to the knowledge bank. The ability to evoke the mountain and tree divas to assist where necessary with the living life and natures changes was emphasised again. More would be revealed when I was given details for the new book I was told.

By the time hands had reached my head, brow and eyes, I could see with inner vision the re-connection of lighted lines between the mind of an individual and their higher mind where guides showed as a matrix of connections. Some will recognise this and some not. I could see that the light stirred and moved to indicate that as the year passes, new connections become operational to reveal greater knowledge and understanding as a result.

At all times the main line or connection to the God consciousness was active, shinning light power and energy to the physical body and its senses, this showed as a picture of a flower unfolding in its bloom, to reveal a central antenna which was the ultimate line or light connection to God himself.

Demonstration of Deep Trance
By Melanie Polley

Evening 16/10/08

At this demonstration of deep trance the child guide Melissa came to talk to us. Full of fun and wit she identified a number of people present by name, those whom she had visited during the week and talked about the various objects that had been moved. Batteries had been drained and certain items gone missing. One or two people were given personal messages relating to their development. Melissa then asked for the Loraine who had been asked to attend to the light switches. She asked for her by surname so identifying the correct person and confirmed that she had been the one responsible for making the lights come on and off when they had been switched off and on.

She then asked for Mrs Pickton so as not to confuse me with the other Jenny present.

'You've been visited by an angel' she asks.
'Yes' I replied. 'I have'
'It was when you were in hospital wasn't it' she said.
'Yes' I replied.
'The medium doesn't know this does she?' Melissa asked.
'No' I said, 'I haven't told her about it'.

'A bloody great big Angel he was'....a pause... 'he held you while you had your operation.'...a pause..... 'He will stay with you while you finish your book'
'Oh' I exclaimed 'Thank you for that confirmation, he was somewhat large as I recall. Thank you so much, Melissa.'

If I ever doubted the existence of Angels I knew I would never again. The healing Angel that I had registered standing at the foot of my hospital bed had shown himself with extremely large wings that seemed to enfold the area containing me. He told me to arise and start living again. He had been directing the nine nuns who were working as teams of three around the clock. They were lined up along my right hand side during the time I had been consumed by the fever of infection after my operation. This had been a turning point in my recovery and was of major significance to me. In the five months since surgery, spirit have been consistently steadfast and true in all their support and communications and have helped me to **hold the light** high.

This lighted presence is now within me shining brightly, as my resolve and confidence, to carry the illumination of the Christ light and his teachings, which have never been so strong. My absolute knowing is no longer a mental holding, but an emotional and mental surety. I have carried out a number of Church services and public demonstrations of clairvoyance and at each event I have become aware of how much closer and stronger is the spirit energy.

I stand in the power and become alight, so that my empty vessel can be filled with the energy of spirit and the dialogue brought forth. For all that I do, is in truth and love as I am driven by an unseen force.

May readers know that all that is printed within this book is written in absolute truth. I stand very much alive having experienced and channelled all that has been formulated into the written words while **Holding the Light**.

Peace and Love to Everyone.

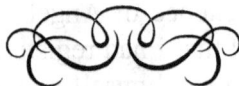

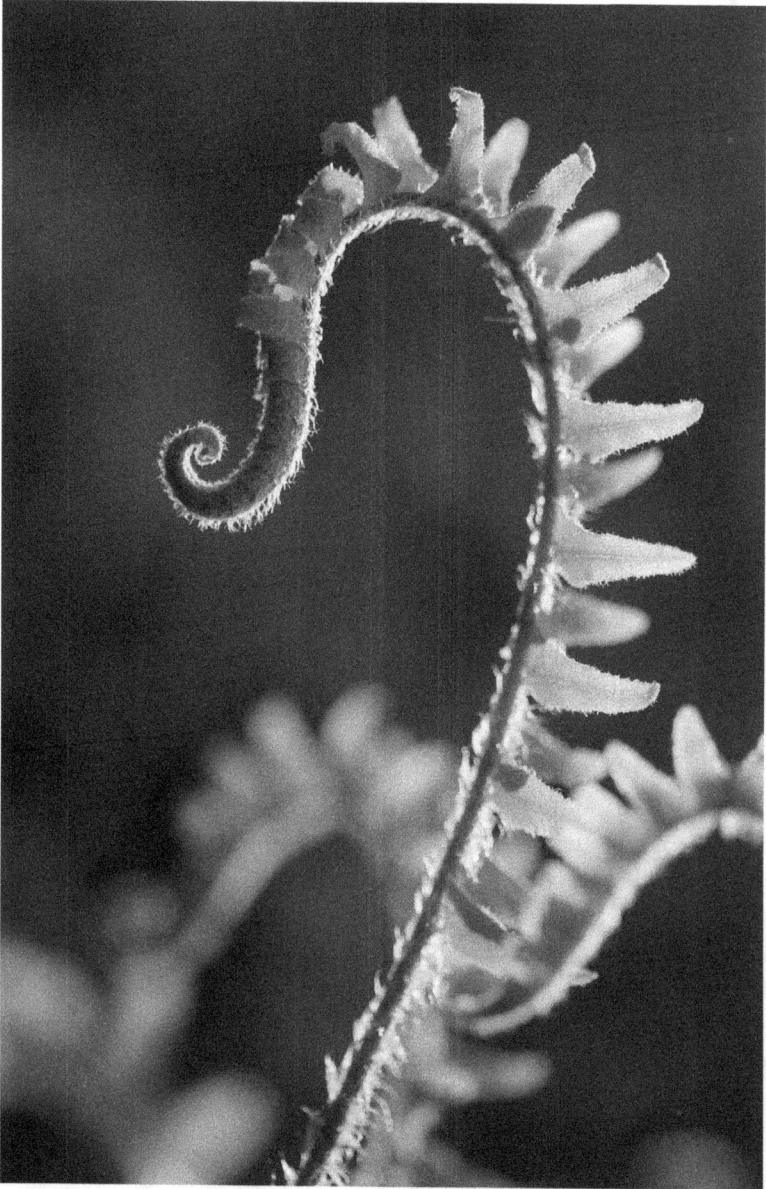

New Creative Growth

Postscript

October 2008

It is now five months after my operation and physically I have mended. My work for spirit continues with a push from those in spirit, 'to get on with the job'. This was made apparent when I attended my local church on Sunday 14th September 2008.

I looked forward to seeing a new medium that was booked for our Sunday Service. I was running late so I didn't have time to change outfits from my casual wear, although I did remember to put on a pearl necklace.

On arrival at the church I found that one of my circle fledgling mediums was chairing the Service and her husband was giving the reading. Her husband is the Vice Chairman of the Church and he was suffering with the beginning of a migraine. Could I give him some healing before the service started? I was asked.

In the back room I gave healing for ten minutes. I left him sitting quietly for a few moments and found his wife in a state of panic as the medium hadn't turned up and it was only two minutes to the start of the service.

'You'll have to do the service she said to me' 'Oh' I said, I'm not exactly dressed for the occasion! 'You look Ok' she said, 'come along'. Suffice to say I took the service that evening without any preparation and it went very well.

At my healing group 'The Healers of All Souls', I have taken up the position of a working healer again and also at the energy centre where therapies are offered. I double up as a healer and reader. It was here that I met again, a lady who was having healing after her cancer treatment.

We had both met when attending as patients and both of us have done well in responding to the healing given during our recovery time.

I have been called upon to give private readings to a number of local people who have been referred to me. In each case there have been connections via friends I know, and an interest shown in healing or personal development.

It seems I am being used as an agent in many areas of interest, relaying information for the education of the novice and the further education of those who are more advanced. Some students need a forum in which to operate, while they consolidate what they know and can do, and then specialise in their chosen area of expertise or extend their present development further.

The circle of new students has assembled and it is a delight to see the enthusiasm of new people whose imaginations have been ignited and whose natural abilities are emerging from absorbing the love and light sent from the world of spirit. When a novice registers the smell of flowers in a room where there are none, you know that spirit is very near. Always that little encouragement is given, to spur us forward in our attempts to discover more.

It is shown to us all, that by **holding the light**, we hold the health and future awakening of humanity within our hands, so it is up to all of us, to do what we can. We are all asked to bring love and peace into the world in which we reside, so others may bask in this Christ light of the Age of Aquarius, and realise the wonder of our own spiritual being in Gods paradise, as it unfolds upon our Earth World.

Eternal Blessings and Peace

Jennifer Pickton

www.ingramcontent.com/pod-product-compliance
Lightning Source LLC
Chambersburg PA
CBHW071223290326
41931CB00037B/1861